CW01558637

Anissa Brodon

Boundaries & Bridges

Parenting Strategies for Abusive Adolescents

Anissa Brodon

Introduction

Parenting an adolescent is one of life's most challenging—and profoundly rewarding—journeys. Yet when our teens turn their frustration, confusion, or hurt into abusive behavior, it can feel like we're caught in a storm with no clear way out. I wrote *Boundaries & Bridges* because I've walked that path—not only as a clinician specializing in family trauma, but also as a mother who has felt the sting of my own child's anger and witnessed the heartbreak that follows. This book is both a map and a compass: it will help you navigate the turbulent waters of abusive adolescent behavior, set sails toward calmer seas of safety, and build bridges back to connection and hope.

Too often, parents find themselves oscillating between harsh discipline and hopeful appeasement, neither of which addresses the root causes of aggression. You may recognize the signs— yelled threats, slammed doors, demeaning words, or even digital harassment—and feel powerless to respond effectively. This cycle breeds guilt, resentment, and isolation on both sides, eroding the very bonds that should sustain your family. Drawing on research in adolescent neurodevelopment and trauma-informed care, along with hard–won lessons from my own household, *Boundaries & Bridges* offers a balanced approach: firm limits paired with compassionate communication, accountability grounded in natural consequences, and restorative practices that honor each person's dignity.

In the chapters that follow, you'll first gain insight into why abusive behavior emerges—how a teen's still-maturing brain, past wounds, and family dynamics converge to produce aggression. You'll learn to set clear, consistent boundaries that protect everyone's safety; implement consequences with calm clarity; and de-escalate high-conflict moments without sacrificing authority or empathy. Then, we'll turn to bridge building strategies: active listening, collaborative problem-solving, therapeutic supports, and resilience-building rituals. Along the way, sample contracts, scripts, and charts will guide you in translating principles into practice. Whether you're facing occasional outbursts or entrenched patterns of abuse, this book will equip you to reclaim peace in your home and nurture the relationship you and your teen both deserve.

Defining "Abusive Adolescent"

Abusive behavior in teens isn't simply bad manners or the occasional outburst; it crosses the line into patterns of aggression and control that harm family members and fracture relationships. When these behaviors become a teen's default strategy for expressing frustration or asserting power, they corrode both individual well-being and the family's sense of safety. In this section, we define the four main forms of adolescent abuse—physical, verbal, emotional, and digital—examine how each manifests, explore the underlying drivers, and outline why it's essential to interrupt these patterns early.

Physical Abuse

Definition & Manifestations

Physical abuse involves any use of bodily force with the intent to intimidate or harm. In adolescents, this can range from shoving, grabbing, or hair-pulling to more violent acts like punching, kicking, or throwing objects. Even seemingly "minor" acts—slaps or harsh pushes—lose their innocuousness when they become repeated tactics for getting attention or dominating family members.

Impact

Safety & Sanctuary

A home should be a haven. Physical aggression transforms it into a battleground, leaving siblings and parents perpetually on guard.

Physical Injury

Bruises, cuts, or sprains may be the most obvious consequences, but repeated low-level violence can cause chronic pain, tension headaches, and long-term musculoskeletal issues.

Emotional Scarring

Victims often internalize the fear and shame of being assaulted by someone they love. This can lead to hypervigilance, anxiety, and difficulty trusting others, including in future romantic or professional relationships.

Underlying Drivers

Impulse Control Deficits

Adolescents' still-developing prefrontal cortex may fail to curb sudden surges of anger, especially under stress.

Learned Behavior

Teens exposed to violence—whether in family, peer, or media contexts—often adopt similar tactics. If hitting was normalized in their environment, they may perceive it as an effective means of solving conflict.

Trauma Reenactment

Teens who have experienced abuse themselves may reenact those patterns, unconsciously exerting power in hopes of avoiding further victimization.

Verbal Abuse

Definition & Manifestations

Verbal abuse encompasses any speech intended to demean, control, or frighten another person. Common forms include:

- **Yelling & Screaming:** Raising one's voice to intimidate or drown out others' attempts to speak.

- **Name-Calling & Insults:** Attaching demeaning labels— "loser," "worthless," "stupid"—to erode self-esteem.

- **Threats:** Warnings of physical violence or emotional withdrawal ("If you ever talk to me like that again, I'll hate you forever").

- **Sarcasm & Belittling Remarks:** Underhanded comments that chip away at someone's confidence over time.

Impact

- **Eroded Trust:** When words become weapons, family members start to anticipate the next verbal attack, curtailing open communication.

- **Low Self-Worth:** Adolescents and parents alike may internalize the negative messages, leading to depression, anxiety, and self-doubt.

- **Interpersonal Damage:** Siblings witness and sometimes adopt these speech patterns, perpetuating a climate of hostility.

Underlying Drivers

- **Emotional Dysregulation:** Teens who struggle to identify or manage their feelings may default to harsh words when overwhelmed.

- **Power Seeks:** Verbal aggression can provide a teen with an immediate sense of control, especially if other areas of life (school, peer relationships) feel chaotic.

- **Identity Formation:** In the throes of forging an identity, some adolescents rebel against parental authority by testing linguistic boundaries, not realizing the cumulative harm of repeated insults.

Emotional Abuse

Definition & Manifestations

Emotional—or psychological—abuse is subtler than physical or verbal forms but arguably more insidious. It involves manipulation and control tactics that undermine a person's emotional health:

- **Gaslighting:** Denying or minimizing events ("That never happened," "You're too sensitive") to make the target question their reality.

- **Withholding Affection:** Purposeful emotional coldness— ignoring, silent treatment, or refusal to engage—used as punishment.

- **Guilt-Tripping & Shaming:** Inducing shame ("I sacrificed everything for you") or guilt ("After all I do, you still treat me this way") to control behavior.

- **Excessive Criticism:** Continual undermining of someone's choices or achievements to foster dependency.

Impact

- **Anxiety & Depression:** Victims often experience chronic worry, feelings of worthlessness, and even suicidal ideation.

- **Attachment Issues:** Repeated emotional manipulation erodes secure bonds, making future trusting relationships difficult.

- **Internalized Negative Beliefs:** Teens may come to believe they are inherently unlovable or defective.

Underlying Drivers

- **Control Needs:** Teens who feel powerless may manipulate others emotionally to regain a sense of agency.

- **Modeling Family Dynamics:** If caregivers or siblings use these tactics, adolescents learn them as "normal."

- **Co-Occurring Mental Health Struggles:** Conditions such as borderline personality traits or chronic low self-esteem can predispose teens to manipulate others emotionally as a way to regulate their own affect.

Digital Abuse

Definition & Manifestations

In an age where screens mediate much of teen life, abuse migrates online:

- **Harassing Texts & DMs:** Bombarding a family member or peer with insults, threats, or demeaning messages.

- **Public Shaming on Social Media:** Tagging someone in humiliating posts or comments designed to embarrass or isolate.

- **Non-Consensual Image Sharing:** Distributing private photos or videos without permission—a legal and emotional violation.

- **Cyberstalking:** Excessive monitoring or surveillance—reading journals, tracking locations, or hacking accounts.

Impact

- **Ubiquitous Threat:** Digital abuse invades every private space—bedrooms, bathrooms—so victims feel unsafe even behind locked doors.

- **Permanent Record:** Once online, harmful content can be difficult to remove, prolonging shame and distress.

• **Peer Reinforcement:** Public audiences (friends, classmates) may join in, amplifying the emotional damage.

Underlying Drivers

• **Anonymity & Distance:** A screen buffer makes it easier to dehumanize the target and escalate abuse.

• **Peer Influence:** Teens often mirror abusive digital norms they see among friend groups or influencers.

• **Impulse vs. Reflection Gap:** Snap judgments and impulsive posting are fueled by the same developmental mismatches that underlie physical and verbal outbursts.

Why Early Intervention Matters

Left unchecked, these four forms of adolescent abuse can harden into adult patterns—affecting academic performance, mental health, and future relationships. Early recognition and targeted intervention can:

• **Prevent Escalation:** Addressing low-level abuse reduces the likelihood of more severe forms emerging.

• **Foster Empathy:** Teaching teens healthier ways to express emotion interrupts cycles of control and shame.

• **Protect Family Well-Being:** Restoring safety and trust in the home environment shields siblings and caregivers from compounding trauma.

Interrupting and Transforming Abusive Patterns

Throughout this book, each chapter will equip you with strategies to:

• **Recognize Warning Signs:** Spot escalating tension before it erupts.

- **Set and Enforce Boundaries:** Establish non-negotiable limits around physical, verbal, emotional, and digital behaviors.

- **Implement Compassionate Consequences:** Use proportional, predictable responses that teach rather than punish.

- **Build Bridges of Empathy:** Cultivate active listening, reflective responses, and restorative "repair talk."

- **Leverage Supports:** Engage therapists, support groups, and community resources when specialized help is needed.

By understanding the full spectrum of adolescent abuse and its roots, you'll be empowered to interrupt harmful patterns, protect your family's sanctuary, and guide your teen toward healthier, more respectful ways of relating.

Goals: Safety, Healing, Reconnection

Before diving into specific strategies and interventions, it's crucial to clarify our north stars. Every principle, tool, and script offered in this book serves one or more of these three interlocking goals: Safety, Healing, and Reconnection. By keeping these end-points in mind, you ensure that every boundary you set, every consequence you apply, and every conversation you have guides your family closer to a stable, compassionate, and connected future.

Safety

A home free from fear is the foundation upon which all other progress rests. Establishing clear boundaries is about more than discipline—it's about creating an environment where every family member can feel secure in body and mind.

Defining Physical Safety

- **Zero Tolerance for Violence:** Physical aggression—hitting, kicking, or throwing objects—must be met with nonnegotiable consequences. These protect victims from harm and signal that violence has no place under your roof.

- **Safe Spaces:** Designate calming zones in your home— corners or rooms where anyone (including you) can retreat when emotions run high. Stock these areas with comforting items (pillows, fidget toys, headphones) and clear instructions for voluntary time-outs.

Ensuring Emotional Safety

- **Predictable Routines:** Consistency in mealtimes, curfews, and check-ins reduces anxiety. When teens know what to expect, they're less likely to react impulsively to uncertainty.

- **Respectful Communication Agreements:** Co-create a family pact that forbids name-calling, threats, and sarcasm. Post it prominently and review it at weekly check-ins so everyone knows the "rules of engagement."

- **Monitoring Digital Boundaries:** In a world where abuse can spill into texts and social media, agree on guidelines for online conduct—no harassing messages, no public shaming, and no sharing private content without consent.

Psychological Safety for Parents

- **Emergency Protocols:** Have a clear plan for serious incidents: a trusted neighbor's number, crisis hotlines, or a safe relative's house. Knowing you have options diminishes helplessness.

- **Parental Time-Outs:** If you feel on the verge of explosive anger, use your own safe space and time-out signal. Modeling self-regulation teaches teens that boundaries apply to all.

By instituting these safety measures, you transform your home from a pressure cooker into a structured refuge—one where trust can be rebuilt because everyone's well-being is guarded.

Healing

Abusive behavior seldom emerges in a vacuum. It often springs from unresolved trauma, overwhelming stress, or unmet emotional needs. Healing acknowledges the underlying pain that fuels aggression.

Trauma-Informed Conversations

- **Empathy Before Evaluation:** Begin tough discussions by acknowledging your teen's feelings: "I know you're angry because you felt unheard." This reduces defensiveness and opens space for reflection.

- **Validated Storytelling:** Invite your teen to share experiences that hurt—past bullying, family conflict, or losses. Listen without interruption, and reflect back what you hear: "It sounds like when you were left out of that game, you felt invisible."

Self-Care as a Family Value

- **Parental Modeling:** Share your own stress-management rituals—journaling, walks, therapy sessions—and explain why they help you stay calm. Teens learn by watching.

- **Family Wellness Practices:** Introduce weekly "wellness moments": a guided breathing exercise after dinner, a short gratitude circle before bedtime, or a Sunday "screen-free" hour to decompress together.

Professional Supports

- **Individual Therapy:** When trauma runs deep—abuse, loss, or severe anxiety—partner with a therapist who specializes in adolescent trauma. Early intervention prevents destructive coping patterns from becoming entrenched.

- **Group Healing:** Support groups for teens (anger-management workshops, peer-mentoring programs) and for parents (caregiver support circles) build community, reduce shame, and offer new perspectives.

Integrating Healing into Boundaries

- **Compassionate Consequences:** Pair firm limits with offers of support—"I know you're upset, but yelling at me still breaks our rule. Once you've completed your time-out, I'll sit with you and help you brainstorm better ways to express frustration."

- **Repair Rituals:** After a conflict, enact a brief ceremony—shared tea, a "reset handshake," or a two-minute apology exchange—so that discipline ends with reconnection, not lingering hurt.

By pairing structure with empathy, you help your teen process pain rather than pass it on—turning moments of conflict into opportunities for growth and emotional resilience.

Reconnection

At the heart of every family lies the desire to belong—to be seen, heard, and valued. Once safety is in place and wounds begin to heal, the real work of rebuilding trust can begin.

Bridge-Building Communication

- **Active Listening Practices:** Set aside devices and distractions. Use open-ended prompts—"Tell me more about that"—and mirror emotions: "It sounds like you felt… when…"

- **"Repair Talk" Templates:** Teach and model the formula: "I feel [emotion] when you [action] because [impact]. Next time, could we [desired change]?" This structured script makes apologies concrete and forward-looking.

Collaborative Problem-Solving

- **Shared Agendas:** Involve your teen in family meetings where everyone lists concerns and brainstorms solutions together. Use voting dots or rank-order exercises to decide priorities fairly.

- **Trial Periods:** When you agree on a new boundary—say, extended curfew—set a two-week trial. Review its success together: "Did this feel fair? What would you tweak?"

Celebrating Connection

- **Ritualized Wins:** Institute weekly "family high-lows," where each member shares one positive highlight and one challenge from the week. This regular ritual reinforces that every voice matters.

- **Shared Projects:** Collaborate on non-family tasks— volunteering, cooking a complex meal, or planning a short outing. These joint ventures shift the relationship from "parent vs. teen" to "team."

Long-Term Partnership

- **Life Mentorship:** As your teen demonstrates maturity, transition from rule-maker to guide—coaching them through budgeting, job interviews, or relationship dilemmas when asked.

- **Evolving Boundaries:** Gradually loosen constraints based on demonstrated responsibility—later curfews, digital freedom, or unsupervised social events—always anchored by check-ins and agreed metrics.

By weaving these reconnection strategies into daily life, you not only repair the rupture caused by abusive behaviors but also fortify a parent-child alliance that can withstand future storms.

Bringing It All Together

Safety, Healing, and Reconnection are not sequential stages but overlapping imperatives. You may revisit safety protocols after a relapse, circle back to healing conversations during high stress, or rebuild bridges even as you reinforce boundaries. Holding these three goals as your guiding stars ensures that your approach never veers into extremes—neither capitulation to abusive behavior nor punitive estrangement. Instead, you offer a balanced path that protects your family while cultivating the empathy, resilience, and mutual respect needed for lasting transformation. As you read on, let these goals anchor every choice you make, every rule you enact, and every word you speak—so that today's challenges become tomorrow's triumphs in your family's journey.

Part I: Foundations

Foundations begin with a clear-eyed understanding of why teens may resort to abusive behavior in the first place. It's not enough to see the outburst and react; we must recognize the brain under construction that fuels impulsivity and emotional volatility. When a teenager's prefrontal cortex is still wiring up its "stop" signals, and their limbic system is driving intense feelings, normal stressors can trigger extreme reactions. Layer onto that any history of trauma, learned patterns from family or media, and emerging mental-health challenges, and you have a perfect storm where hurting others feels like the only way to regain control. By grasping these neurological and psychological roots, parents can respond with informed empathy rather than merely escalating conflict.

Equally critical is mapping the family system itself—the invisible web of roles, rules, and routines that silently shapes every interaction. Who in your home steps into the rescuer's shoes? Who carries the brunt of blame? Are peacemaker habits enabling a cycle where harmful behavior is swept under the rug? When we chart these dynamics, we see where abusive patterns gain their foothold: perhaps an argument is always "solved" by giving in, or a teen's anger goes unchecked because avoidance appears easier than confrontation. Recognizing whether your household tends toward enmeshment, triangulation, or boundary erosion is the first step to redesigning a system that empowers rather than enables.

Ultimately, the foundation of change rests on the parent's own self-awareness and resilience. Setting firm boundaries with a calm, grounded presence means knowing your personal hot buttons and practicing the very self-regulation you demand of your child. It also means prioritizing your own well-being—building a support network, carving out time for rest and reflection, and celebrating small wins when moments of progress emerge. In the crucible of family conflict, a parent's steady commitment to growth not only models healthier coping but plants the seeds for genuine transformation: turning a home once marked by fear into one defined by safety, respect, and mutual understanding.

Chapter 1: Understanding Abusive Behavior in Teens

Understanding abusive behavior in adolescence is more than an act of rebellion—it's a signal that something deep within a teen's development, environment, or lived experience has gone awry. To effectively address and transform these behaviors, parents must first peer into the underlying mechanisms driving them. In this chapter, we'll explore the developmental architecture of the teen brain, examine the key risk factors that tip frustration into aggression, and learn how to distinguish garden-variety defiance from patterns of true abuse.

The teenage brain is a work in progress, with the "accelerator" of emotion—the limbic system—maturing well before the "brakes" of planning and impulse control in the prefrontal cortex. This natural imbalance makes adolescents prone to intense, rapid mood swings and impulsive reactions. When stress mounts—whether from academic pressure, social turmoil, or family conflict—their still-immature neural wiring can misfire, converting ordinary frustration into explosive outbursts. Recognizing this biological backdrop helps parents respond with informed patience rather than punitive frustration.

Yet biology is only part of the story. Trauma, whether experienced firsthand or witnessed in the home or community, primes a young mind to interpret the world as threatening. Teens who have seen aggression modeled—by caregivers, peers, or media—learn that force is an acceptable problem-solving tool. Co-occurring mental health struggles (anxiety, depression, ADHD) further lower the threshold for aggressive impulses. And environments marked by chaos, instability, or unstructured free time sap coping resources, making destructive behaviors more likely.

Finally, not all defiance equates to abuse. A slammed door, a sharp retort, or a missed curfew can be typical rites of passage. But when patterns of intimidation—physical, verbal, emotional, or digital—become a teen's go-to strategy for control, the behavior crosses into abuse. In the pages ahead, we'll unpack how to spot these red-flag patterns early, interrupt the cycle before it takes hold, and guide your adolescent toward healthier ways of asserting independence.

Adolescence represents one of the most dramatic periods of human brain development, marked by both incredible growth and significant pruning of neural connections. During this time, two primary systems—the limbic system and the prefrontal cortex—mature at different rates, creating a natural imbalance between emotion and regulation. Understanding this developmental landscape is crucial for parents of challenging teens: it dispels assumptions of willful cruelty and reframes outbursts as predictable, if still unacceptable, reactions to life's pressures.

The Limbic System (Emotion Engine)

The limbic system, anchored by the amygdala, is the brain's emotional command center. In early adolescence, this network matures rapidly:

- **Heightened Sensitivity to Reward:** Teens experience pleasure more intensely than children or adults. A compliment from a peer or the adrenaline of a risky stunt floods the brain with dopamine, reinforcing thrill-seeking behaviors.

- **Peer Approval Priority:** Neural circuits attuned to social evaluation become hyperactive. A single dismissive glance or offhand remark from friends can feel devastating, triggering defensive or retaliatory responses.

- **Emotional Overdrive:** The amygdala's quick-fire threat detection means ordinary stressors—criticism from a parent, a disappointing grade—can register as urgent dangers, prompting

19

fight-or-flight reactions before the "thinking" brain can intervene.

This emotional engine propels adolescents toward novel experiences and social bonds but also makes them vulnerable to extreme mood swings. Parents witnessing sudden surges of anger, fear, or joy can feel as though their teen is "out of control," unaware that their child's brain is simply operating on overdrive.

The Prefrontal Cortex (Control Center)

In contrast, the prefrontal cortex — the seat of planning, judgment, and impulse inhibition — develops on a slower timeline:

- **Protracted Pruning and Myelination:** Throughout adolescence and into the mid-twenties, the brain strengthens frequently used neural pathways and prunes away underused ones. Myelination (insulation around neurons) increases signal speed, but this process is gradual.

- **Emerging Executive Functions:** Skills such as weighing long-term consequences, multitasking, and resisting temptations are rooted in prefrontal development. Early teens may struggle with delaying gratification ("I know I have homework, but I really want to finish this game now").

- **Delayed Integration with Limbic System:** The prefrontal cortex only gradually gains authority over the limbic system. Until the "brakes" catch up to the "accelerator," teens can be hijacked by emotion faster than they can marshal reasoned responses.

Because these control centers are still under construction, adolescents often act on impulse. A minor frustration — being asked to unload the dishwasher, for instance — can trigger an outsized reaction: slamming doors, shouting, or even physical aggression. It's not that they choose cruelty; their neural hardware simply isn't fully equipped to modulate strong emotions under stress.

Bridging the Developmental Gap

Awareness of this imbalance empowers parents to respond more effectively:

- **Compassionate Limits:** Rather than viewing outbursts as deliberate defiance, frame them as neural mismatches. State boundaries calmly: "I know your feelings are intense right now, but hitting isn't allowed. Let's take a break and talk when we're both calmer."

- **Skill-Building Opportunities:** Use calm moments to teach regulation techniques—deep breathing, counting to ten, or brief physical activity—to help teens practice engaging their control centers.

- **Predictable structure:** Regular routines and clear expectations reduce uncertainty, lowering the limbic system's threat perception and giving the prefrontal cortex more space to operate.

By honoring the teen brain's unique architecture—an emotion engine revving ahead of its braking system—parents can replace frustration with empathy, firmness with flexibility, and punishment with coaching. This developmental lens transforms a parent's role from "enforcer of rules" to "guide in growth," laying the groundwork for healthier, more regulated adulthood.

Risk Factors: Trauma, Modeling, Mental Health, Environment

While the neurodevelopmental stage of adolescence creates a predisposition for impulsive reactions, whether a teen's frustration erupts into abusive behavior often depends on a constellation of risk factors—some rooted in past experiences, others present in daily life. By understanding how trauma, modeling, mental health challenges, environmental stressors, and even parental alienation interact with a developing brain, parents can target interventions where they'll have the greatest impact.

Trauma

Teens who have endured violence, neglect, or significant loss often learn to view aggression as a form of self-protection or a means of reclaiming control. A teenager who witnessed domestic violence, for instance, may believe that force guarantees safety, replaying those patterns when they feel threatened. Unresolved trauma leaves the nervous system on constant alert—hyper-vigilant to perceived slights—so even a casual criticism from a teacher or a sibling's teasing can trigger an outsized, defensive response. Standard disciplinary tactics often fail in these cases because the behavior is driven less by rebellion than by survival instinct. Trauma-informed therapies—such as EMDR, trauma-focused CBT, or somatic approaches—help teens process painful experiences, integrate memories, and develop healthier coping strategies, reducing the perceived need to resort to aggression.

Modeling

Behavior is profoundly shaped by what adolescents observe. If a young person sees caregivers, older siblings, or influential peers resolving conflicts through intimidation, yelling, or manipulation, those tactics become normalized as effective means to an end. Media portrayals of "strong" figures who dominate through force further blur the line between assertiveness and abuse. To counteract harmful modeling, parents must become deliberate exemplars of respectful conflict resolution: using calm tones, engaging in active listening, and employing "repair talk" after mistakes. Encouraging participation in activities—like team sports, debate clubs, or peer-led mediation programs—exposes teens to alternative strategies and role models who embody empathy and cooperation.

Mental Health

Underlying psychological conditions frequently intensify irritability, lower frustration tolerance, and fuel impulsivity—fertile ground for abusive outbursts. ADHD can manifest as chronic restlessness and difficulty delaying gratification; depression often brings persistent irritability and hopelessness; anxiety heightens sensitivity to rejection; and emerging personality disorders may foster manipulative or explosive patterns. Without timely diagnosis and treatment, these issues not only exacerbate conflict but can also alienate the teen from supportive relationships. Early screening by a qualified mental-health professional is vital. When indicated, evidence-based interventions—medication management, DBT skills training, or family-based therapy—equip adolescents with concrete tools for emotional regulation, distress tolerance, and effective interpersonal communication.

Environment

Chronic stressors in a teen's surroundings can deplete even the most resilient coping mechanisms. Academic pressures—from high-stakes exams to heavy workloads—create relentless tension. Community violence or neighborhood instability reinforce the notion that aggression is necessary for survival. Even within the home, chaotic schedules, unpredictable rules, and irregular routines can undermine a teen's sense of security. Parents can mitigate these risks by establishing consistent daily rhythms—regular meals, predictable bedtimes, and clear expectations—and by limiting exposure to violent media. Introducing family-wide stress-reduction practices—such as evening walks, weekend mindfulness exercises, or creative outlets—replenishes emotional reserves and models healthy self-care.

Parental Alienation

Parental alienation occurs when one caregiver manipulates the teenager to turn against the other parent, often through denigration, guilt-tripping, or withholding love. This dynamic fractures loyalty, breeds confusion, and can catalyze aggressive behaviors aimed at the "favored" parent. Teens caught in the crossfire may lash out physically or verbally as they struggle to exert control over their fractured attachments. To counter alienation, parents must shield their teen from triangulation: maintain a united front on boundaries, avoid negative talk about the other parent, and seek family therapy or parenting coordination when necessary. Rebuilding trust involves transparent communication, reinforcing the teenager's right to love both parents, and modeling cooperative co-parenting even amid conflict.

By pinpointing which of these five risk factors most strongly influences your teen—trauma, modeling, mental health, environment, or parental alienation—you can tailor your approach: trauma-informed therapy for deep wounds; intentional positive modeling to replace harmful scripts; psychiatric evaluation and skill-building for mental-health concerns; environmental adjustments to reduce chronic stress; and co-parenting strategies to undo alienation. This targeted strategy maximizes the chance that interventions will interrupt the trajectory from frustration to abuse, guiding your adolescent toward healthier ways of coping and relating.

Differentiating "Typical Teenage Rebellion" vs. Abuse

Adolescence is a natural crucible for boundary-testing. Teens push against limits to discover who they are and where they belong. A slammed door, a missed curfew, or a sharp retort can feel dramatic—but may simply be rites of passage rather than red flags. Yet when these behaviors harden into patterns of intimidation, control, or hurt, they cross the line from "normal" rebellion into abuse. Recognizing the difference is critical: mislabeling defiance as abuse can damage trust, while treating abuse as mere rebellion leaves families vulnerable to harm. Below are three key criteria—frequency & pattern, intent & target, and impact on the household—to help you distinguish garden-variety defiance from behavior that requires specialized, safety-first interventions.

Frequency & Pattern

- **Typical Rebellion:** Occasional, situation-specific acts of defiance. Examples include staying out past curfew after a special event, rolling eyes during a family lecture, or skipping a chore when feeling overwhelmed. These incidents tend to be isolated, short-lived, and often accompanied by remorse once consequences kick in.

- **Abusive Behavior:** Recurring, escalating tactics aimed at instilling fear or asserting control. This might look like weekly verbal tirades loaded with threats ("If you tell me to do that one more time, I'll ruin your stuff"), repeated digital harassment of siblings, or physical intimidation by blocking doorways or shoving. The common thread is consistency and escalation: each episode builds on the last, forming a recognizable strategy rather than a one-off lapse.

Why It Matters: A single late night or heated argument is unlikely to erode family safety. But patterns of aggression condition everyone to expect—and accommodate—abuse, normalizing it until walls of fear spring up around ordinary interactions.

Intent & Target

- **Typical Rebellion:** Primarily an expression of frustration, curiosity, or a bid for independence. Teens vent their irritation at "the rules" ("I just hate this curfew!") or test limits ("Let's see if they really mean no phone after 9 PM"). The focal point is the boundary itself, not a deliberate desire to harm another person.

- **Abusive Behavior:** Deliberate actions designed to undermine another's dignity or sense of safety. Physical threats ("I'll punch you if you don't stop"), name-calling ("You're a worthless idiot"), or digital shaming (posting siblings' private moments online) are aimed squarely at people, not merely at rules. The abuser's objective is control—forcing others to capitulate or cower.

Why It Matters: Misunderstanding intent can lead to misdirected responses. Addressing rebellious teens as though they mean to hurt cultivates resentment, while ignoring the malicious intent behind abusive acts leaves victims unprotected and perpetrators unaccountable.

Impact on the Household

- **Typical Rebellion:** Family members feel annoyed, disappointed, or frustrated, but rarely unsafe. After the storm passes, relationships rebound quickly: chores resume, apologies are made, and normal routines continue.

- **Abusive Behavior:** Creates a pervasive climate of fear or guardedness. Siblings may avoid certain rooms to escape verbal attacks; parents might hesitate to enforce rules, knowing the teen could retaliate. Joy and spontaneity erode, replaced by hyper-vigilance and emotional distance.

Why It Matters: The hallmark of abuse is its corrosive effect on family well-being. If daily life revolves around damage control, consent when asking for chores, or tip-toeing around volatile moods, you're dealing with more than teenage defiance — you're living in a high-risk environment that demands immediate, specialized intervention.

Shifting to Safety-First Strategies

Once behavior crosses into sustained aggression with the aim of harm or control, it's time to pivot from ordinary disciplinary tactics to safety-first protocols. Standard responses — grounding, lectures, scolding — can backfire against an abuser, who may escalate in retaliation. Instead, specialized approaches focus on:

- **Protecting Targets:** Separating vulnerable family members, establishing clear "safe zones," and ensuring victims know how to seek help.

- **Interrupting Patterns:** Using early-warning systems to halt rising tension, deploying de-escalation scripts, and applying predictable, proportional consequences.

- **Building Accountability:** Engaging teens in repair talk, requiring them to articulate the impact of their actions, and involving them in restorative practices that rebuild trust.

In the next chapter, we'll dive into concrete boundary-setting techniques — how to design rules that leave no ambiguity, enforce them with compassion, and maintain your own equilibrium when conflicts flare. By distinguishing rebellion from abuse — and responding accordingly — you'll protect your family's safety while teaching your adolescent healthier ways to express needs, assert autonomy, and manage emotions.

Chapter 2: The Psychology of the Family System

In every household, unseen currents of roles, rules, and relationships shape how members interact—especially under stress. When abusive behavior emerges in an adolescent, it rarely springs from one person alone; it's entangled in the larger family ecosystem. Understanding these dynamics gives parents the power to rewire unhelpful patterns and foster healthier connections. In this chapter, we'll explore how informal roles take root, why some parental responses enable rather than empower, and how to spot—and interrupt—the cycle of abuse before it spirals out of control.

Family Roles and Dynamics

Families unconsciously assign roles to help manage conflict and maintain stability. One child may become the "hero," excelling academically or behaviorally to compensate for turmoil elsewhere. Another might slip into the "scapegoat" role, blamed for tensions that actually stem from deeper issues. Parents themselves can fall into complementary parts—"rescuer" swooping in to solve problems, or "enforcer" meting out harsh discipline. While these roles may offer temporary order, they also lock everyone into rigid patterns that perpetuate conflict. A scapegoat teen, for example, learns that acting out guarantees attention, while a rescuer parent unwittingly reinforces abusive tactics by stepping in to shield the teen from consequences.

Enabling Versus Empowering Patterns

When confronted with abusive behavior, it's natural to want to stop the conflict quickly—yet quick fixes often enable more abuse. Enabling looks like bailing a teen out of natural consequences ("I'll tell your teacher you were sick"), capitulating to threats ("Fine, you can skip chores if you stop screaming"), or avoiding discussions to keep the peace. Empowerment, by contrast, means holding firm to boundaries while teaching skills for independence. An empowering parent might say, "I understand you're angry about chores. Chores still need doing—let's plan a time that works for you," and then follow through on agreed consequences when rules are broken. Over time, empowerment builds the teen's capacity for self-regulation and accountability.

Cycle of Abuse: Recognition and Intervention

Abusive family dynamics often follow a predictable four-phase loop:

- **Tension Building:** Small irritations—snide comments, slammed doors—mount unaddressed.

- **Incident:** A verbal tirade, physical shove, or digital attack erupts.

- **Reconciliation:** Apologies, promises to change, and temporary calm ensue.

- **Calm:** A lull before simmering feelings ignite the next cycle.

To interrupt this loop, intervene both before and after incidents. During tension-building, use de-escalation tools—time-outs, calm reminders of rules, or a shift in setting. After reconciliation, resist letting apologies erase accountability; instead, reinforce the need to rebuild trust through consistent, respectful actions. By mapping roles, choosing empowerment over enabling, and breaking the cycle of abuse at multiple points, families can transform patterns of aggression into pathways for growth and connection.

Family roles and dynamics

Families are living systems, complete with implicit rules, norms, and roles that guide behavior without ever being written down. These informal roles help everyone find a place—and, under stress, they often crystallize into rigid patterns that perpetuate dysfunction. When an adolescent begins exhibiting abusive behavior, it cannot be understood in isolation; it is woven into this broader tapestry of family dynamics. Below, we unpack four archetypal roles—the Hero, the Scapegoat, the Rescuer, and the Lost Child—and illustrate how they interact to sustain a self-reinforcing system. By mapping these patterns, parents can identify leverage points for change and reassign roles in healthier ways.

The Hero

Who they are: The Hero child excels—academically, athletically, or socially—and often assumes the task of keeping the family's reputation intact. Their successes become a buffer against turmoil, as achievements distract from underlying tensions.

How the role forms: In families under stress, praise may come only when someone performs exceptionally. A teen who brings home straight A's or shines in sports receives adult admiration, momentarily deflecting attention from conflicts or crises elsewhere in the household.

Impact on the family:

- **Surface Harmony:** The Hero's wins create a facade of normalcy—holiday dinners are planned around their recital; family photos highlight their trophies.

- **Sibling Resentment:** Brothers and sisters may feel invisible or undervalued, breeding jealousy that can morph into their own acting-out behaviors.

- **Hero Pressure:** The Hero child internalizes immense expectation. The fear of failure can lead to anxiety, perfectionism, or secretive struggles away from prying eyes.

Path to change: Acknowledge achievements without using them to paper over problems. Encourage the Hero to share feelings about family stress, modeling that success and vulnerability can coexist.

The Scapegoat

Who they are: When tensions rise, the Scapegoat absorbs blame. Their misbehavior—skipping school, defiance, or aggression—focuses attention on them, diverting scrutiny from deeper issues.

How the role forms: Parents or siblings may project guilt and anxiety onto one child to avoid confronting their own conflicts. A teen reacting to parental discord becomes the evident "problem," allowing caregivers to feel momentarily competent by "fixing" that one issue.

Impact on the family:

• **Temporary Relief:** Addressing the Scapegoat's behavior— punishing them, seeking therapy—gives the illusion of progress.

• **Entrenched Shame:** The Scapegoat internalizes the message: "Something is wrong with me." Chronic guilt, low self-esteem, and acting-out behaviors escalate.

• **Systemic Stagnation:** As long as the Scapegoat remains the focus, systemic dysfunction goes unexamined and unaddressed.

Path to change: Broaden the lens beyond individual misbehavior. Engage the family in exploring triggers for conflict and distribute responsibility for solutions across all members, not just the labeled child.

The Rescuer

Who they are: Often a parent or older sibling, the Rescuer rushes in to solve problems—shielding the abuser from consequences or smoothing over arguments to restore peace.

How the role forms: Motivated by compassion or fear of escalation, Rescuers intervene prematurely: negotiating extensions on curfews, covering up for broken rules, or mediating conflicts without letting parties express grievances.

Impact on the family:

- **Enabling Tactics:** The abuser learns that threats or outbursts guarantee intervention, reinforcing abusive strategies.

- **Parental Burnout:** Constant crisis management exhausts Rescuers, who carry the weight of responsibility for everyone's emotions.

- **Victim Silencing:** True victims of abuse—siblings or the parent targeted by the teen—may feel unheard as the Rescuer monopolizes attention.

Path to change: Rescuers must practice restraint: allow natural consequences to unfold, step back during minor conflicts, and coach family members in resolving disputes rather than resolving them for them.

The Lost Child

Who they are: Quiet, withdrawn, and conflict-averse, the Lost Child retreats from family drama, avoiding both praise and blame.

How the role forms: When tension spikes, this child learns that staying invisible reduces the risk of being caught in crossfire. Silence becomes a survival strategy.

Impact on the family:

- **Unchecked Power:** The abuser faces little resistance from the Lost Child, reinforcing a sense of dominance.

- **Emotional Isolation:** Loss of connection prevents the Lost Child from processing feelings, increasing risk of depression or social anxiety.

- **Hidden Needs:** Their needs go unmet because they neither ask for help nor draw attention to themselves.

Path to change: Gently invite participation—assign small, supported roles in family tasks or meetings. Validate their contributions, creating a safe space for expression.

Rewiring the System

These four roles interact in a feedback loop: the Hero distracts, the Scapegoat absorbs blame, the Rescuer intervenes, and the Lost Child withdraws—each reinforcing the others. To transform this system:

- **Map Roles Publicly:** In a neutral family meeting, chart who tends to fill each role and how it affects everyone.

- **Rotate Responsibilities:** Give each member opportunities to step into different roles—e.g., the Hero practices vulnerability, the Scapegoat leads problem-solving, the Rescuer steps back, and the Lost Child voices opinions.

- **Establish New Norms:** Co-create family agreements that reward collaboration over enabling, curiosity over blame, and inclusion over withdrawal.

By illuminating hidden dynamics and intentionally reassigning roles, families can break free from dysfunctional patterns—creating space for healthier connections, shared accountability, and collective resilience.

Enabling vs. empowering patterns

When families confront an adolescent's abusive behavior, two contrasting dynamics often emerge: enabling, which inadvertently reinforces aggression, and empowering, which fosters accountability and growth. Recognizing these patterns is essential: while enabling may restore temporary calm, it perpetuates abuse by rewarding it. Empowering, by contrast, shifts the dynamic from "power over" to "power with," teaching teens to regulate emotions, solve problems, and respect boundaries.

Enabling

Quick Fixes

In an effort to quell immediate tension, parents may bargain with abusive teens:
"If you stop yelling now, I'll let you skip tonight's chores."
Though this halts the outburst, it sends a clear message: aggression is an effective strategy for getting what you want.

Conflict Avoidance

To sidestep uncomfortable confrontations, families might ignore low-level verbal attacks—snide comments or sarcasm—hoping the behavior will fade on its own. Over time, these unchecked slights escalate, signaling to the teen that they can push boundaries without consequence.

Overprotection

Well-meaning parents often "rescue" teens from the fallout of their own actions: paying fines for a car scratch caused in anger, calling teachers to excuse missed assignments, or replacing broken devices. While intended to shield the teen from hardship, these interventions deprive them of vital lessons in responsibility and natural cause-and-effect.

Consequences of Enabling

Reinforced Aggression: Teens learn that disrespect or intimidation reliably yields relief or rewards.

Eroded Accountability: Without facing logical outcomes, adolescents fail to develop self-regulation and problem-solving skills.

Parental Burnout: Constant crisis management exhausts caregivers emotionally and physically, reducing their capacity for consistent boundary enforcement.

Empowering

Collaborative Boundary-Setting

Instead of dictating rules unilaterally, involve your teen in co-creating household guidelines. Use open-ended questions:
"Which behaviors make you feel unsafe at home? How should we respond if those happen?"
When teens contribute to rule design—curfew times, screen-time limits, or respectful communication protocols—they're more likely to honor agreements they've helped craft.

Natural Consequences

Allow outcomes to flow logically from actions:

- A missed curfew means waiting until the next weekend for outings.

- A smashed phone goes unrepaired until the teen uses allowance money to fix it.
  These real-world consequences tie behavior directly to results, fostering accountability.

Skill-Building

Replace punitive measures with coaching moments:

- **Emotional Regulation:** Practice deep-breathing exercises or use a stress journal to name and process feelings before they erupt.

- **Problem-Solving Frameworks:** Teach steps—define the issue, brainstorm solutions, weigh pros and cons, select an approach, and review outcomes.
  Over time, teens internalize these tools, reducing reliance on external enforcement.

Benefits of Empowerment

- **Agency and Ownership:** Teens develop confidence as they see their choices directly shape their freedoms.

- **Mutual Respect:** Collaborative processes level the power dynamic, promoting respectful dialogue over coercion.

- **Resilience and Growth:** Facing natural outcomes and practicing self-management builds skills that extend far beyond the family realm.

Shifting the Dynamic

Transitioning from enabling to empowering requires intention and consistency:

- **Audit Your Responses:** Over a week, note whenever you intervene to rescue or placate. Reflect on alternative empowering responses you could offer.

- **Communicate Intent:** Explain the shift to your teen: "I want you to learn how to solve problems and handle consequences—that's how you become independent."

• **Set Transitional Supports:** Initially, you might lower stakes —shorten grounding periods or offer guided problem-solving sessions—to ease into natural consequences.

• **Celebrate Efforts:** Acknowledge each time your teen uses a regulation technique or participates in boundary-setting. Positive reinforcement cements new habits.

By replacing quick fixes and overprotection with collaboration, logical outcomes, and skill coaching, you move your family from a crisis-management mode to a growth-oriented partnership. Empowerment not only curbs abusive behavior but equips your adolescent with the self-control, empathy, and problem-solving abilities needed for healthy adult relationships.

Interrupting the Cycle

Abusive family dynamics often spin in a familiar loop: tension builds, an incident erupts, apologies follow, and calm returns— only for tensions to mount again. Without targeted interventions, this cycle can persist indefinitely, each turn chipping away at trust and safety. The good news is that by applying strategies at both the tension-building and reconciliation phases, families can flatten the peaks of conflict, shorten the cycle's duration, and gradually rewire interactions toward respect and connection.

Pre-Incident Interventions

Notice Early Warning Signs

The first step is spotting the subtle cues that tension is rising. A teen's raised voice, clenched jaw, rigid posture, or restless pacing often heralds an impending outburst. Parents should also attend to their own physiological signals—flushed skin, rapid heartbeat— that indicate they too are on the brink of reactivity.

Offer a Brief Pause

When you recognize these warning signs, invite a short break before conflict escalates. A simple script works well:

"I can see we're both getting heated. Let's take five minutes apart to calm down, then come back and talk."

This pause gives the limbic systems time to cool and the prefrontal cortices a chance to reengage, reducing the likelihood of impulsive aggression.

Use a Pre-Agreed De-Escalation Signal

Establish a neutral cue—perhaps the word "pause" or a raised hand—that either party can deploy when feeling overwhelmed. Because the signal is agreed upon in advance, it carries clear permissions: the conversation stops, no guilt or argument ensues, and both sides honor the break.

Post-Incident Accountability

Hold to Agreed Consequences

Apologies are important, but they don't erase the need for accountability. If your family contract specifies that a physical shove costs two hours of extra chores, enforce that outcome even after your teen has said "I'm sorry." Consistency here teaches that trust is rebuilt through actions, not just words.

Debrief the Episode

Once emotions have cooled and consequences applied, schedule a brief debrief—ideally within 24 hours. Use open-ended questions to guide reflection:

"What do you think sparked your outburst?"

"How did you feel in that moment?"

"What might you try next time to express yourself without crossing the line?"

This structured conversation strengthens self-awareness and helps your teen practice identifying triggers and alternative responses.

Reinforce Genuine Progress

Positive change deserves recognition. When your teen uses the "pause" signal, completes a consequence without complaint, or applies a new coping skill, acknowledge it specifically:

"I noticed you suggested a break before things got heated—that showed real growth."

Such reinforcement accelerates the formation of healthier habits and underscores the family's commitment to mutual respect.

Looking Ahead

With a clear view of your family's invisible architecture—roles that entrench abuse, patterns that enable it, and cycles that perpetuate it—you're now prepared to redesign your household's foundation. You've learned to spot early tension, hit pause before emotions overflow, hold everyone to fair accountability, and celebrate progress when it occurs. These insights form the launchpad for Part II, where we'll translate analysis into action: setting clear, consistent boundaries that protect safety; crafting compassionate consequences; and building the empathic bridges that reconnect your family. By moving thoughtfully from insight to implementation, you'll cultivate a home environment defined by safety, healing, and reconnection—one intentional step at a time.

Chapter 3: Your Role as a Parent

Parenting an abusive adolescent is as much an inward journey as it is an outward challenge. Before you can guide your teen toward healthier behaviors, you must first understand the internal forces shaping your own responses. **Self-awareness** begins with identifying your triggers—the specific words, tones, or actions that consistently push you from calm into frustration or anger. Notice the physical cues—tightened shoulders, a racing heart— and the thoughts that follow ("How dare they speak to me like that?"). Behind these triggers lie deeply held **beliefs** about respect, obedience, and parental authority. Reflect on where those convictions originated—your upbringing, cultural norms, or personal values—and ask whether they serve your current goal of fostering mutual respect. Finally, get clear on your own **boundaries**: what behaviors you will not tolerate and why. When you know your limits, you can communicate them calmly and enforce them consistently, without being hijacked by guilt or reactivity.

Sustaining the energy and clarity required for this work hinges on **parental self-care** and the strength of your **support network**. You cannot pour from an empty cup. Carve out daily rituals— whether a brief walk after dinner, ten minutes of journaling before bed, or a weekend hobby—that rejuvenate your mind and body. Prioritize sleep, regular movement, and balanced nutrition to keep stress hormones in check. Equally vital is cultivating relationships with trusted friends, family, or fellow parents who understand your journey. Share victories and frustrations in these circles without fear of judgment; simply knowing you're not alone replenishes resolve. Consider professional outlets too—whether a therapist who helps you unpack family-of-origin wounds or a support group for caregivers of challenging teens, external perspectives can offer fresh strategies and hold you accountable to your own needs.

Even with self-awareness and self-care in place, standing firm on boundaries requires **resilience**—the capacity to remain grounded amid storms of conflict. Cultivate a **growth mindset**, viewing setbacks not as failures but as data points guiding your next approach. Celebrate every incremental win—your teen's apology, a calm de-escalation, or a day without abusive incidents —as proof that change is possible. Anchor yourself in purpose by regularly revisiting your deeper "why": protecting safety, teaching respect, and nurturing your teen's potential. Practice **calm presence** techniques—deep breathing, brief pauses before responding, or silently counting to five—to interrupt reactive cycles. Over time, these habits strengthen your emotional endurance, model the self-regulation you expect from your teen, and transform you from a reactive disciplinarian into a steady, empathetic leader capable of steering your family toward healing and lasting change.

Self-awareness: triggers, beliefs, boundaries

Before you can set healthy limits for your teen, you must first understand your own emotional landscape. This self-awareness lays the groundwork for consistent, calm boundary enforcement and helps you respond thoughtfully rather than reactively when conflicts arise.

Identify Your Triggers

Begin by cataloging the specific words, tones, and actions from your teen that reliably push your buttons. Maybe it's that sharp edge in their voice when they say, "You don't understand me," or the way they roll their eyes after you ask them to complete a chore. Tune in to the physical cues in your body—your jaw tightening, heart rate accelerating, stomach knotting—and notice the thoughts that flood your mind ("How dare they talk to me like that!" or "They're so disrespectful"). For one week, keep a private "trigger journal": each time you feel a strong emotional spike, jot down the situation, your bodily reaction, and your immediate thought. Over time, patterns will emerge. Naming these triggers builds a crucial buffer between stimulus and response: the moment you recognize a trigger, you gain the space to take a breath, collect your thoughts, and choose a more measured reaction.

Examine Underlying Beliefs

Triggers often stem from deeply held beliefs about parenting, obedience, and respect. Perhaps you grew up in a household where children were expected to obey without question, so any challenge to your authority feels like a personal affront. Or you may carry the conviction that showing emotion equals weakness, leading you to clamp down harder when you sense vulnerability. Reflect on where these convictions originated—your own childhood experiences, cultural or religious norms, or formative mentors—and evaluate whether they still serve your goals. Ask yourself: Does the belief "A child must always obey" foster a respectful relationship, or does it teach my teen to comply only when fear of punishment is greater than the urge to rebel? By questioning and, if necessary, reframing these core beliefs, you free yourself from unconscious drivers of reactivity and open the door to more compassionate, effective parenting strategies.

Clarify Your Boundaries

Boundaries are not arbitrary edicts but clear statements of what you will and will not tolerate. Drawing on your trigger journal and belief reflections, define your nonnegotiables in precise, behavior-based terms. For example:

- "I will not allow yelling that includes name-calling."

- "I will not permit any form of physical intimidation—no pushing, no grabbing."

- "I will not engage in discussions where one person shouts over the other."

Write these boundaries down and refine the language until each statement feels clear and enforceable. When boundaries are anchored in your own self-awareness—knowing exactly which behaviors push your limits and why—you can communicate them calmly: "I hear you're upset, but calling me names crosses the line. We'll take a five-minute break and resume when we're both calmer." More importantly, clarity lets you follow through consistently. When your teen tests these limits, you can remind them of the agreed boundary and apply the predetermined consequence without second-guessing yourself or getting sidetracked by guilt.

By identifying your personal triggers, examining the beliefs that fuel them, and clarifying your own boundaries, you transform from a reactive disciplinarian into a reflective, grounded guide. This inner work empowers you to set limits that feel authentic and sustainable—creating a household environment where rules are predictable, respect is mutual, and both you and your teen can navigate conflict with greater confidence and care.

Importance of parental self-care and support network

Parenting an abusive adolescent demands extraordinary emotional stamina. You're not only guiding a teen through volatile behaviors but also managing your own reactions, fears, and stresses. Attempting this work without replenishing your reserves is a recipe for burnout—leaving you depleted and less able to provide the calm authority your teen needs. Just as flight attendants tell us to put on our own oxygen masks before assisting others, you must practice consistent self-care and build a strong support network. These two pillars—daily restoration practices and nourishing relationships—work together to sustain your patience, clarity, and resilience.

Daily Restoration Practices

Small, intentional rituals can serve as daily lifelines when you're parenting in crisis. Because time is scarce, these practices should be brief, non-negotiable, and embedded into your routine:

- **Ten-Minute Walks After Dinner:** A short stroll around the block lets you transition from the day's demands into evening downtime. The combination of fresh air, gentle exercise, and rhythmic movement helps lower cortisol levels and reset your stress response.

- **Deep-Breathing Breaks Before Bed:** Spend two to five minutes lying or sitting quietly, inhaling deeply for a count of four and exhaling for a count of six. This practice engages the parasympathetic nervous system, signaling to your brain that it's safe to unwind.

- **Five-Minute Journaling Sessions:** Keep a small notebook by your bedside or kitchen counter. Jot down your toughest moment of the day—and one thing you're grateful for. This simple exercise shifts focus from problems to progress, reinforcing a balanced perspective.

By treating these rituals as appointments with yourself—blocking them on your calendar or linking them to existing habits like brushing your teeth—you reduce the chance of skipping them when stress peaks. Over time, these micro-pauses accumulate, replenishing your emotional reserves and preventing the chronic fatigue that undermines effective parenting.

Nourishing Relationships

Isolation magnifies stress, making every conflict feel more personal and inescapable. Cultivating nurturing relationships with people who understand your struggle is vital:

- **Trusted Friends and Relatives:** Identify two to three individuals—perhaps a close friend, a sibling, or a parent—who can listen without judgment. Schedule regular check-ins, whether a weekly phone call or a monthly coffee date, to share both victories ("My teen used our de-escalation signal today!") and frustrations ("We had a meltdown over chores again"). Simply articulating these experiences reduces emotional load and reminds you that you're not alone.

- **Fellow Parents:** Seek out other caregivers facing similar challenges—through school parent groups, community centers, or online forums. Exchanging practical tips ("Here's how I introduced a family meeting") and offering mutual encouragement fosters solidarity. Hearing that another parent overcame comparable obstacles can reignite hope during bleak moments.

These connections serve as both sounding boards and emotional anchors, buffering you against self-doubt and reinforcing your commitment to change.

Professional and Peer Support

While peer empathy is invaluable, sometimes specialized guidance is necessary. Don't hesitate to enlist professional and structured peer support:

- **Support Groups for Parents of Troubled Teens:** Many community mental-health centers and nonprofit organizations host groups where parents learn evidence-based strategies, share resources, and hold one another accountable. The structured nature of these groups ensures that you receive curated insights rather than ad-hoc advice.

• **Family Therapists or Parenting Coaches:** A trained therapist or coach can help you identify blind spots—perhaps an overreliance on enabling behaviors or a blind spot around your own triggers. They can introduce tailored techniques for boundary-setting, de-escalation, and self-regulation. Regular sessions provide a safe space to process your emotions, refine strategies, and track progress.

• **Online Workshops and Webinars:** When in-person options are scarce, virtual courses on topics like trauma-informed parenting, adolescent brain development, or conflict resolution can expand your toolkit. Many courses include moderated discussion boards, offering a hybrid of professional and peer support.

Investing in these formal supports underscores the seriousness of your commitment—not just to your teen's transformation but to your own well-being. It's not self-indulgence; it's strategic reinforcement that enables you to serve your family more effectively.

Parenting an abusive adolescent is an endurance test, demanding compassion, consistency, and emotional fortitude. By embedding daily restoration practices into your life and cultivating a robust network of personal and professional support, you ensure you have the energy, clarity, and resilience to meet each challenge with calm authority. Remember: You cannot pour from an empty cup. Prioritizing your well-being is not a detour from parenting—it's the path that makes sustainable, transformative parenting possible.

Building resilience in yourself to stand firm

With self-awareness and self-care laying the groundwork, the next step is cultivating the resilience that lets you uphold boundaries calmly and consistently—even when your teen pushes back. Resilience is not innate; it's a muscle you build through intentional practices that reframe setbacks, reinforce purpose, and sustain momentum. Below are four strategies to deepen your inner strength and become the stable anchor your family needs.

Adopt a Growth Mindset

Resilient parents view challenges as opportunities to learn rather than as personal failures. When a consequence doesn't stick or a conversation derails, ask yourself: *What can this teach me?* Instead of thinking, "I failed to enforce the rule," reframe that moment as data: "My teen reacted strongly—perhaps I need to adjust the timing or clarify the expectation." Keep a brief "reflection log" where you note one insight per conflict: what went well, what didn't, and one tweak for next time. Over weeks, you'll see patterns and improvements. This iterative process transforms frustration into fuel, keeping you flexible, hopeful, and better equipped to meet each new challenge.

Anchor in Purpose

On tough days, the immediate heat of conflict can obscure the broader vision. Strengthen your resolve by regularly reconnecting with your "why": the core reasons you set boundaries in the first place. Maybe it's to ensure physical and emotional safety, to teach respect, or to guide your teen toward healthier adult relationships. Craft a concise affirmation—"I set limits so my home stays safe and respectful"—and place it somewhere visible: on your bathroom mirror, the fridge door, or your phone screensaver. Each time you pause to read it, you evoke the deeper values driving your actions. This ritual refocuses your energy on long-term goals rather than short-term discomfort.

Celebrate Small Wins

Sustainable change emerges through countless incremental victories. Too often, parents and teens alike overlook modest progress because it doesn't match a dramatic breakthrough. Instead, intentionally acknowledge every positive step:

- Your teen paused when you signaled "time-out."

- You delivered a consequence without raising your voice.

- A previously volatile topic was navigated calmly.

Record these wins in a shared "success jar" or a simple checklist. At week's end, review the list—celebrate with a family high-five or a small treat. Recognizing effort, not just perfection, boosts confidence and reinforces that new patterns are possible. Each celebration becomes a building block for greater resilience.

Practice Calm Presence

True authority is grounded in composure, not coercion. When conflict arises, anchor yourself with a moment of calm: take three slow, deliberate breaths; press your feet into the floor; soften your shoulders. Then speak in a level tone, using concise, behavior-focused language: "We agreed no name-calling. Let's pause for five minutes." Avoid lecturing or rehashing past grievances—focus on the present boundary and its consequence. Your calm presence models the emotional regulation you want your teen to learn. Over time, they'll mirror this steadiness, reducing the intensity of future clashes.

By deepening self-awareness, honoring your own needs, and nurturing these resilience practices, you become the composed leader your family needs. This inner work not only empowers you to enforce boundaries with empathy and consistency but also demonstrates for your teen the very skills—reflection, adaptability, and perseverance—that will serve them throughout life. In the next section, we'll translate this fortified stance into concrete boundary-setting techniques and collaborative bridge-building exercises to guide your family's journey toward safety, healing, and reconnection.

Part II: Boundaries

Part II of this book marks the transition from theory to practice. After laying the groundwork by understanding why adolescents may resort to abusive behavior, we now focus on the concrete steps you can take to reshape dynamics at home. Boundaries are not about punishment—they're about clarity. When everyone knows the "rules of the road," there's less room for confusion, fear, or resentment. In these chapters, we'll explore how to define what's acceptable in your household, how to communicate those expectations in ways that resonate with teens, and how to ensure that rules feel fair rather than arbitrary.

Once you've established clear limits, the next challenge is enforcing them with consistency and compassion. Consequences should flow naturally from the misbehavior—think grounding for missed curfews or requiring repair chores for broken items—so your teen learns the real-world price of their actions. But we also recognize that adolescents are experts at pushing boundaries and testing resolve. That's why Part II also delves into de-escalation techniques and "repair scripts" you can use when tensions flare. You'll practice delivering consequences calmly, avoiding power struggles, and restoring peace without sacrificing your authority.

Finally, boundaries are not set in stone. As your teen grows and demonstrates maturity, those limits will need to evolve. Part II closes by showing you how to revisit and adjust rules collaboratively, ensuring that your family's framework remains both protective and empowering. By mastering these boundary-setting strategies, you'll create a home environment where respect replaces fear, cooperation replaces coercion, and every member— from parent to adolescent—knows exactly where they stand.

Chapter 4: Setting Clear, Consistent Limits

Boundaries are the structural beams that support a healthy family home—especially when parenting an adolescent whose behavior has veered into aggression. Without clear, consistent limits, everyone lives in uncertainty: parents guess which rules will stick, and teens test invisible lines until someone gets hurt. Establishing well-defined boundaries transforms this chaos into a predictable framework where expectations are transparent, consequences are reliable, and mutual respect can flourish.

Clear limits do more than prohibit unwanted behavior; they create a container of safety and trust. When an adolescent knows exactly what actions trigger a response—whether it's raising a fist, shouting a slur, or sending harassing texts—they feel contained within a reliable system. This predictability reduces anxiety. Parents worry less about hidden traps or sudden escalations, and teens can navigate daily life knowing the "rules of the road." Over time, this shared understanding reinforces the belief that the household is governed by fairness rather than capricious whims, laying the groundwork for cooperation rather than rebellion.

Consistency is the bedrock of effective boundary-setting. A rule enforced only sporadically—or worse, arbitrarily—undermines the entire structure. If a teen is grounded after a physical outburst one week but excused with a warning the next, they learn that boundaries are negotiable and that testing limits will eventually pay off. Conversely, when every violation of an agreed-upon rule consistently results in the stated consequence, adolescents internalize that actions have predictable outcomes. This consistency is not about rigidity or cruelty; it's about reliability. A parent's calm certainty in following through delivers a powerful message: "I mean what I say, and you can trust that I will follow through."

Crafting boundaries requires intentionality and clarity. Broad, abstract edicts like "Be respectful" or "Stop misbehaving" leave too much room for interpretation. Effective limits focus on concrete, observable behaviors—"No name-calling," "Keep your hands to yourself," or "No posting images of family members without permission." By tying rules to specific actions, you eliminate debates over intent and semantics, making enforcement straightforward and fair.

In the chapters to follow, we will explore how to define boundaries that align with your teen's developmental stage, involve them in co-creating the household contract, and design consequences that educate rather than punish. We will also delve into strategies for maintaining your own calm presence when enforcing limits and repairing relationships when conflicts arise. By mastering the art of setting clear, consistent limits, you'll provide your adolescent with the structure they need to thrive— and your family with the stability and trust that make true healing possible.

The function of boundaries in safety and trust

Boundaries serve as the guardrails of family life, preventing destructive "crashes" and guiding everyone toward predictable, acceptable behavior. In a household with an adolescent prone to explosive outbursts, ambiguity around limits only fuels anxiety and conflict: Is raising one's voice "yelling"? Does one sarcastic jab count as verbal abuse? Without clear parameters, teens may test the limits until something breaks—a dish, a relationship, or both. When boundaries are explicitly defined and reliably enforced, these dilemmas vanish. Everyone knows exactly where the line is drawn, reducing the guesswork that often sparks power struggles.

Reducing Ambiguity and Hidden Loopholes

Imagine a rule labeled simply "No yelling." What qualifies as yelling? Is speaking loudly during excitement off-limits? Or are only aggressive tones prohibited? By detailing acceptable and unacceptable levels of volume and tone—"Raising your voice to express excitement is fine; using a harsh tone or shouting insults is not"—you eliminate gray areas. Similarly, spelling out that "one insult still breaks our rule against name-calling" closes loopholes: your teen learns that abuse isn't a game of semantics. These precise definitions act like high-visibility road signs, steering everyone away from dangerous behavior before it escalates.

Building Trust Through Consistency

Trust is the currency that lubricates family interactions. When you say, "We'll pause for ten minutes if voices get too loud," and then follow through every time, your word gains weight. Conversely, if you threaten consequences but back down when pushback arises, your teen learns that boundaries are mere suggestions, encouraging further testing. Consistent enforcement makes your expectations credible: your adolescent learns that "this is what happens, every single time," and adjusts behavior accordingly. Over weeks and months, this consistency transforms distrust into confidence. Parents grow less anxious—knowing the boundaries will hold—and teens experience relief in a structured environment where the rules are unchanging and the outcomes predictable.

Creating Emotional Safety

Physical safety is fundamental—no one should fear being struck, shoved, or physically blocked in their own home. Yet emotional safety is equally vital. When boundaries protect against verbal and emotional abuse—insults, threats, sarcasm, gaslighting—family members can speak and act without the dread of unseen landmines. Boundaries such as "No name-calling, even in anger" or "No silent treatment as punishment" reassure everyone that their dignity and feelings are respected. In such an atmosphere, a teen who feels anger rising can safely express frustration ("I'm upset because I thought you said I could go") without fearing the conversation will spiral into humiliation or retribution.

Fostering Mutual Predictability

The magic of clear boundaries lies in their reciprocal nature: they apply equally to all family members. When parents model the same limits—speaking calmly even when angry, owning mistakes without excuses—they demonstrate fairness and mutual accountability. This mutual predictability nurtures respect: teens recognize that "Mom and Dad don't get special exceptions," and parents see that "My teen follows the same rules I do." In turn, this shared contract of behavior stabilizes the home environment, reducing the emotional whiplash that comes from capricious rule changes or uneven enforcement.

Anchoring Respect and Empowerment

Firm yet fair boundaries send a powerful message: "I respect you enough to make my expectations clear, and I trust you to meet them." This approach contrasts sharply with arbitrary or punitive rule-making, which breeds resentment and rebellion. Instead, boundaries become tools of empowerment. Teens learn the life skills of self-regulation, delayed gratification, and ethical decision-making within the safe constraints of the family system. As they demonstrate reliability, parents can confidently grant incremental freedoms—later curfews, unsupervised outings, expanded digital privileges—knowing that the established guardrails will guide responsible choices.

By understanding and applying the function of boundaries—reducing ambiguity, enforcing consistency, ensuring emotional safety, fostering mutual predictability, and anchoring respect—you create a household where both parents and adolescents feel secure, understood, and empowered. This environment of predictable limits and reliable follow-through lays the groundwork for deeper healing, genuine trust, and lasting connection.

Crafting age-appropriate, behavior-based rules

Not all rules suit every age or personality. Rules that feel arbitrary or disconnected from daily life breed confusion and resentment. To maximize buy-in and effectiveness, ground your household guidelines in observable behaviors, tailor their complexity to your teen's developmental stage, involve them in crafting the rules, and keep the list short—focused on the most pressing concerns. Below, we unpack four principles for designing rules your adolescent can understand, own, and honor.

Start with Behaviors, Not Personas

Abstract expectations—"Be respectful," "Act mature"—sound noble but leave too much to interpretation. Instead, specify concrete actions:

- "Speak without name-calling or threats." Defines verbal respect in precise terms.

- **"Keep hands to yourself."** Clearly prohibits physical aggression.

- "Use 'I feel…' statements when addressing conflicts." Guides both tone and structure of communication.

- "Address family members by name without profanity." Outlines respectful address.

By focusing on discrete behaviors, you eliminate ambiguity. Everyone knows exactly what actions are permitted—and which cross the line. This clarity makes it easier to enforce rules calmly and consistently, and reduces arguments over "What did I do wrong?"

Match Complexity to Developmental Stage

Adolescents' cognitive and emotional capacities evolve rapidly. Align rule complexity with their maturity:

- **Younger Teens (11–14):** Bright-line rules work best. Their prefrontal cortices are still developing, so concrete, simple directives minimize misinterpretation:

  - **Example:** "No hitting or pushing, ever."

  - **Why It Works:** There's no room for debate—physical aggression is off-limits in all circumstances.

- **Older Adolescents (15–18+):** Capable of nuanced thinking, they can handle layered guidelines that acknowledge gray areas:

  - **Example:** "No belittling comments in front of siblings; if you disagree, start with 'I feel… because…'"

  - **Why It Works:** This rule teaches conflict resolution skills, modeling mature communication while still prohibiting harmful behavior.

- **Individual Tailoring:** Beyond age, consider personality and experience. A teen with impulse-control challenges might need shorter, clearer rules; a highly verbal teen can benefit from more elaborate communication protocols.

Collaborate Where Possible

Co-creating rules with your teen turns directives into agreements. Collaboration fosters ownership, reducing power struggles:

- **Set the Stage:** Choose a neutral time and place—perhaps a weekend afternoon at the kitchen table.

- Ask Guided Questions:

  - "What behaviors make you feel unsafe or disrespected at home?"

  - "How do you think we should respond if that happens?"

  - "Which rules will help you feel trusted and supported?"

- **Brainstorm Together:** Let ideas flow freely. Encourage your teen to voice concerns and suggest rules.

- **Evaluate and Refine:** Discuss each proposal's fairness and feasibility. Ask, "Will this rule be easy to remember? What's a logical consequence if it's broken?"

- **Document the Agreement:** Write down the final rule list, add it to your family command center, and let both parent and teen sign.

When teens see their suggestions incorporated, they feel respected and are more motivated to abide by the household contract.

Limit the Number of Rules

A sprawling rulebook dilutes focus and makes consistent enforcement difficult. Instead:

- **Identify Top Priorities:** Choose three to five behaviors that pose the greatest risk or tension in your home—physical aggression, verbal abuse, digital harassment, property damage, or habitual defiance.

• **Keep It Manageable:** Fewer rules mean clearer communication and stronger follow-through. When a rule is broken, it's easier to point to one clear violation rather than sift through a dozen possible infractions.

• **Rotate as Needed:** As progress is made, retire or revise rules. Introduce new ones only when truly necessary.

Bringing It All Together

By centering rules on observable behaviors, matching their complexity to your teen's developmental stage, collaborating in their creation, and keeping the list concise, you craft a framework your adolescent can understand—and follow. These measures not only curb abusive behaviors but also model clear communication, mutual respect, and shared responsibility. With well-designed, behavior-based rules serving as your family's roadmap, both you and your teen can navigate conflicts confidently—and grow together in safety and trust.

Consequence design: natural vs. imposed

Consequences are the educational engine of boundary enforcement—they teach cause and effect, helping adolescents internalize responsibility for their actions. When consequences mirror the misbehavior ("natural") or are applied thoughtfully by caregivers ("imposed"), they reinforce that every choice carries a predictable outcome. Below, we explore both approaches, their advantages, and how to blend them into a balanced system of accountability.

Natural Consequences

Definition & Examples

Natural consequences occur when the outcome flows logically from the teen's own behavior, without parental invention. For instance:

- If a teen throws their phone in anger and breaks it, the device remains unusable until they pay to repair or replace it.

- If a student skips study time and then performs poorly on a test, they face the grade they earned—without parental intervention to "fix" it.

Advantages

- **Perceived Fairness:** Because the result arises organically, teens view it as a direct, just response rather than arbitrary "punishment."

- **Clear Cause-and-Effect:** The linkage between behavior and outcome is unambiguous, reinforcing the lesson that personal actions drive real-world results.

- **Reduced Parental "Punisher" Role:** Parents avoid being seen as the enforcer of discomfort, instead allowing life itself to teach the lesson.

Limitations

Natural consequences aren't always feasible: broken phones may be under warranty, test grades may feel insufficiently corrective, or some outcomes could pose safety issues if left entirely "natural" (e.g., allowing a teen to skip medical follow-up).

Imposed Consequences

Definition & Examples

When natural outcomes are delayed, insufficiently instructive, or potentially harmful, parents impose logical, behavior-linked consequences. Examples include:

- **Grounding** a teen from social activities after a physical aggression incident.

- **Suspending privileges** such as gaming, car use, or outings following repeated boundary violations.

Guidelines for Effective Imposed Consequences

- **Proportionality:** Scale the consequence to the severity of the misbehavior. A harsh shove might warrant a two-day grounding; a minor insult might merit a same-day family chore.

- **Immediacy:** Apply the outcome as close in time as possible to the rule violation—ideally within hours, not days—so the connection remains vivid.

- **Predictability:** Before enforcement, ensure your teen understands exactly which behaviors trigger which consequences. Posting a simple "Behavior → Consequence" chart helps eliminate uncertainty.

Advantages

- **Flexibility:** Allows parents to address situations where natural outcomes fall short.

- **Structure:** Demonstrates that household rules are backed by consistent follow-through, reinforcing trust in the system.

Blending Both Approaches

A hybrid model often yields the strongest learning. For instance, if a teen engages in digital harassment of a sibling, you might:

• **Impose** a temporary social-media blackout—immediate, proportional, and predictable.

• **Invoke** a natural consequence by requiring the teen to draft and deliver sincere apology letters or messages to each target, restoring relationships through direct action.

This blended strategy leverages the immediacy of imposed consequences and the authenticity of natural outcomes, deepening the teen's understanding of both accountability and empathy.

Best Practices for Delivering Consequences

• **Communicate Calmly and Briefly:** In the heat of the moment, state the rule, remind your teen of the pre-agreed consequence, and follow through—no lectures or emotional pressure.

• **Maintain Consistency:** Every infraction triggers the same outcome, reinforcing that boundaries aren't negotiable.

• **Reinforce Growth:** When your teen accepts a consequence without argument or applies a new coping skill, acknowledge it: "You handled that calmly today and followed through with your chore—that's real responsibility."

By understanding how boundaries underpin safety and trust, tailoring rules to your teen's age and specific behaviors, and designing consequences that educate rather than merely punish, you'll transform your household into a structured—but still loving—environment. This balance of natural and imposed outcomes lays the groundwork for deeper healing, cooperation, and ultimately, the bridge-building work to come in Part III.

Chapter 5: Implementing Consequences with Compassion

When boundaries are crossed, consequences serve as the bridge between behavior and understanding, illustrating that actions carry real-world outcomes. Yet, the effectiveness of this learning mechanism hinges not on severity, but on delivery. Consequences delivered with harshness or unpredictability often backfire— eroding trust, fueling resentment, and even exacerbating the very abusive behaviors you aim to curtail. Implementing consequences with compassion, by contrast, preserves your teen's dignity, reinforces your connection, and models the respectful communication you wish to cultivate.

Compassionate consequence-setting begins with **calm, clear communication**. In the heat of conflict, emotions can surge, and parents may feel compelled to lecture or vent frustrations. Instead, frame your response in neutral, behavior-focused language: "When you pushed me, it broke our rule against physical aggression. As agreed, you'll have two hours of extra chores." Briefly stating the rule, naming the behavior, and invoking the predetermined outcome cuts through emotional reactivity and centers the exchange on cause and effect rather than blame.

Sidestepping **power struggles** is the next crucial element. Adolescents are primed to resist control, especially when they feel cornered or shamed. Rather than issuing ultimatums—"Do your chores now or you're grounded for a week!"—offer structured choices: "You can start your chores now and be done by dinner, or do them tomorrow morning before school—but they do need to get done." This approach maintains your boundary while granting your teen agency, reducing defiance and opening space for cooperative problem-solving.

Perhaps the most vital pillar of compassionate enforcement is **consistent follow-through**. Empty threats and inconsistent application teach teens that boundaries are negotiable—encouraging them to test and exploit loopholes. When you follow through calmly and reliably, you earn credibility and build your teen's confidence in the system. Consistency also helps normalize consequences, reducing the drama surrounding rule enforcement. A predictable response—applied every time a rule is broken—gradually shifts family dynamics from crisis management to steady, respectful order.

Finally, compassionate consequences conclude with **repair and reflection**, not lingering resentment. After the consequence is served, plan a brief "debrief" conversation when emotions have cooled: "What do you think triggered your outburst? How might you handle it differently next time?" This restoration phase reinforces learning, fosters empathy, and preserves relational warmth.

In this chapter, we will delve deeper into the scripts, strategies, and mindset shifts that enable parents to implement consequences with empathy and authority. You'll discover how to communicate firmly yet kindly, defuse power struggles before they ignite, maintain unwavering consistency, and close disciplinary episodes with healing conversations. By mastering these skills, you'll transform consequences from punitive punishments into compassionate coaching moments—guiding your adolescent toward accountability, self-regulation, and enduring respect.

Communicating Consequences Calmly and Clearly

Delivering consequences effectively hinges on the way you communicate them. When boundaries are crossed, your tone and language can either reinforce respect and understanding—or unintentionally escalate the conflict. The following principles will help you convey outcomes with clarity, neutrality, and compassion, transforming disciplinary moments into opportunities for growth rather than power struggles.

Use Neutral Language

Emotional or judgmental phrasing puts teens on the defensive and obscures the real issue. Instead of:

"You're so disrespectful—I'm done with you!"

Opt for a neutral, behavior-focused statement:

"When you called me names just now, it crossed our agreed boundary. As discussed, you'll lose screen time for the next 24 hours."

Why Neutral Language Works

• **Minimizes Reactivity:** Stripping out words like "disrespectful" or "stupid" prevents your teen from feeling personally attacked.

• **Keeps Focus on Behavior:** Naming the specific action— calling names—clarifies exactly what is unacceptable.

• **Reinforces Contractual Ground:** Reminding your teen of the prior agreement ("As discussed…") underscores that this is not a surprise punishment but a predictable outcome.

Practical Tips

• Before speaking, take a deep breath and consciously drop any emotionally charged words.

• Use "When…then…" constructions to link behavior and consequence: "When you [behavior], then you [consequence]."

• Speak in a steady, even tone—neither loud nor whispered.

Stick to the Facts

Avoid narratives, moral lectures, or condescending asides. Your message should simply outline the observed behavior and the agreed consequence:

"You hit your sister. That action breaks our rule against physical aggression. Your consequence is an extra hour of chores this week."

Why Factual Statements Work

• **Eliminates Subjectivity:** Stating exactly what happened—hitting your sister—prevents disputes over interpretation.

• **Reduces Drama:** Focusing on the fact rather than the emotion keeps the exchange concise and prevents spiraling.

• **Models Objectivity:** Demonstrates how to discuss conflicts without blaming or shaming, a skill your teen can emulate.

Practical Tips

• Use simple past-tense verbs to describe what you saw: "You threw," "You said," "You blocked."

• Reference the specific rule broken: "We agreed no physical aggression."

• Name the consequence clearly and briefly: "You'll do an extra hour of chores this week."

Keep It Brief

Long-winded lectures rarely change behavior; they only prolong the conflict. Aim for a concise delivery of two to three sentences:

• **State the behavior:** "When you slammed the door…"

- **Invoke the rule:** "…it broke our agreement to handle anger calmly."

- **Announce the consequence:** "You'll take a 30-minute room time-out."

Then pause. Allow your teen space to absorb the information. If they have questions or push back, invite them to revisit the discussion later:

"I know this feels unfair. Let's talk more about it after dinner when we're both calm."

Why Brevity Works

- **Maintains Clarity:** A short message is easier to understand and less likely to be misremembered.

- **Prevents Escalation:** Fewer words mean fewer opportunities for emotional triggers.

- **Respects Processing Time:** Teens often need moments to shift from reactive to reflective mindset.

Practical Tips

- Prepare your core message mentally before speaking.

- Resist the urge to justify or explain excessively during the heat of the moment.

- Use a calm closing phrase—"Let's pause here and revisit later if needed"—to signal the conversation's end.

Affirm the Relationship

Consequences should correct behavior, not erode the parent-child bond. End with a statement that separates the action from your love and your hopes for your teen:

"I care about you, and I want you to learn healthier ways to express anger. Let's talk tomorrow about what triggered you and how we can handle it differently next time."

Why Affirmation Works

- **Preserves Dignity:** Reminds your teen they are valued, even when their actions aren't.

- **Keeps the Door Open:** Signals that you're invested in understanding and supporting them beyond punishment.

- **Models Empathy:** Demonstrates how to combine accountability with care—a critical life skill.

Practical Tips

- Use "I" statements to own your feelings: "I feel worried," "I care about you."

- Offer a specific plan for reconnection: scheduling a time to talk or share a meal.

- Avoid vague reassurances; tie your affirmations to concrete actions: "We'll talk tomorrow at breakfast."

By using neutral language, sticking to observable facts, keeping your delivery concise, and affirming your relationship, you communicate consequences—calmly and clearly—so your teen understands both the behavior's impact and your continued support. This compassionate approach transforms discipline into a collaborative learning process, reinforcing boundaries while nurturing trust and respect.

Avoiding Power Struggles and Emotional Reactivity

When conflicts flare with an abusive teen, it's natural for emotions to surge on both sides—yet matching intensity with intensity only fans the fire. Avoiding power struggles and managing your own reactivity is critical for preserving authority, modeling self-regulation, and steering interactions back toward problem-solving. Below are four strategies—maintaining calm physiology, using "I" statements, offering choices within limits, and resisting the bait—that work in tandem to defuse tension and uphold boundaries with dignity.

Maintain a Calm Physiology

Your body often speaks before your words. If you enter a confrontation already tense—shoulders hunched, breath shallow, pulse racing—you're primed to sound sharp and move abruptly, triggering your teen's fight-or-flight reflex. Instead, practice a quick three-breath reset before responding:

1. **Inhale slowly** through your nose for a count of four.

2. **Hold** for a count of one.

3. **Exhale** gently through your mouth for a count of six.

Repeat three times while consciously dropping your shoulders and relaxing your jaw. This physiological shift sends signals to your brain that it's safe to lower the volume—both literally and figuratively. Your voice will naturally soften, your posture open, and your facial expressions more composed. By modeling this self-regulation, you demonstrate the very skill you want your adolescent to learn: the ability to pause, breathe, and respond thoughtfully rather than react impulsively.

Use "I" Statements

Blame-laden language ignites defensiveness. Labeling your teen as "out of control" or "spoiled" wounds their sense of identity and escalates conflict. "I" statements, by contrast, focus on the impact of the behavior and invite empathy:

- **I feel…** ("I feel unsafe")

- **When you…** ("When you shoved me")

- **Because…** ("Because I worry that someone could get hurt.")

Full example:

"I feel unsafe when you shove me because I could fall and get injured. We need to use words instead of hands."

This formula separates the person from the action and clarifies why the behavior matters. It also shifts the dialogue from accusation to partnership: you're expressing concern for both of you, not attacking their character. Over time, "I" statements cultivate mutual respect and reduce the emotional charge that fuels power struggles.

Offer Choices Within Limits

Ultimatums—"Do your chores now or no computer all week!"—set up win-lose scenarios that invite defiance. Instead, present structured options that maintain firm boundaries while preserving your teen's sense of agency:

"You have two choices: start your chores now and finish by dinner, or do them tomorrow morning before school. Either way, the chores need to be done."

This approach accomplishes three goals:

- **Empowers decision-making:** Teens who feel some control over how they comply are likelier to choose cooperation over rebellion.

- **Keeps focus on the outcome:** The boundary (chores get done) remains non-negotiable; only the timing is flexible.

- **Reduces confrontational energy:** A choice avoids the zero-sum fight of parent vs. teen.

For more complex issues—like digital misuse—you can scale options (e.g., shorter social-media access now vs. supervised use later), always tying choices back to the core boundary.

Don't Take the Bait

Abusive teens may escalate or redirect blame to trigger your emotional reaction: "You never listen!" or "You're ruining my life!" Responding in kind just deepens the conflict. Instead, use a two-step technique:

Acknowledge the emotion:

"I hear your frustration."

Reiterate the boundary and consequence:

"The rule is no name-calling. Today's consequence is the agreed 24-hour loss of screen time."

This concise structure keeps the exchange on track: you validate the feeling without conceding the behavioral standard. If needed, offer to revisit the conversation later when both are calmer:

"I know you're upset. Let's take a break and talk again in 30 minutes."

Putting It All Together

Avoiding power struggles and emotional reactivity isn't about suppressing your own feelings; it's about managing them to maintain authority and connection. By resetting your physiology, using "I" statements, providing structured choices, and refusing to be baited into shouting matches, you preserve your teen's dignity and model the emotional control you expect from them. Over time, these techniques build a culture of respect rather than coercion—an environment where boundaries are upheld not by force, but by shared understanding and self-regulation.

Following Through: Consistency as the Bedrock

Consistency is the cornerstone of effective boundary enforcement. Without reliable follow-through, even the clearest rules lose meaning. Your teen must learn that agreements are not mere suggestions but the framework that ensures safety and respect in your home. The following practices will help you cement consistency and turn consequences into trusted signposts rather than arbitrary punishments.

Apply Consequences Immediately

The power of a consequence lies in its immediacy. When the interval between misbehavior and outcome stretches beyond hours —or worse, days—the link weakens in your teen's mind. Whenever possible, impose the agreed consequence within minutes or hours of the infraction:

- **Example 1:** If your teen shouts a profanity at dinner, they lose smartphone privileges for the remainder of the evening.

- **Example 2:** When a teenager refuses to unload the dishwasher after reminders, they handle dishes exclusively for the next two meals.

This prompt application leverages the recency effect in learning: the brain more readily connects the behavior with its consequence. It also prevents the resentment that builds when teens perceive that parents only act on their own schedule rather than in direct response to the behavior.

Honor Every Agreement

71

Boundaries are contracts of trust. If you declare, "No video games for two days," enforce it without exception. A single "get-out-of-jail" card teaches your teen that testing limits yields leniency. Instead, maintain unwavering follow-through:

- **No Exceptions:** Even on special occasions—vacations, weekends, or family celebrations—stick to the consequence schedule.

- **Consistent Voice:** When asked for an exception, calmly restate the rule: "We agreed two days; we'll stick to that."

Honoring every agreement demonstrates reliability. Your teen learns that "if you break the rule, this precise outcome follows every single time," which instills respect for boundaries and discourages repeated violations.

Document Agreements

For recurring issues, a posted list of rules and their associated consequences removes ambiguity and keeps expectations front and center. Create a simple chart:

Behavior	Consequence
Physical aggression	24-hour loss of screen time
Name-calling or threats	Two extra hours of chores
Missing curfew without notice	One-evening grounding

Place this chart in a high-traffic area—on the fridge or near the family calendar—so everyone sees it daily. Documentation:

- **Eliminates Memory Gaps:** Both parent and teen can reference the chart rather than relying on recall.

- **Reduces Disputes:** When "But you didn't say that!" arises, you can point to the posted agreement.

Over time, this visual cue reinforces that the system is stable, transparent, and fair.

Acknowledge Compliance

Consequences aren't solely about correction; they're also about reinforcing positive behavior. When your teen accepts a consequence without argument or completes it promptly, offer genuine praise:

"I noticed you finished your extra chores without complaint. That shows real responsibility."

Acknowledgment serves three functions:

- **Positive Reinforcement:** It rewards the behavior you want to see—compliance and accountability.

- **Relationship Repair:** It reminds your teen that your connection isn't defined solely by conflict.

- **Motivation Booster:** Recognizing effort makes your teen more likely to repeat the positive action.

Keep acknowledgments specific and sincere, focusing on the teen's choice rather than your relief.

Review and Adjust as Needed

Consistency doesn't mean rigidity. If a particular consequence consistently fails to deter the behavior—or feels disproportionately harsh—collaborate with your teen to revise it. For example:

- **Too Mild:** If a one-hour grounding isn't curbing repeated aggression, extend to a day or add a natural consequence (repairing damaged items).

- **Too Harsh:** If losing all electronics for a week leaves your teen isolated and defiant, shorten the duration or swap in a natural consequence.

Schedule periodic family check-ins to review how rules and consequences are working. Ask:

- "Are the outcomes fair and effective?"

- "Which rules feel too strict or too loose?"

- "What adjustments would help you learn from mistakes?"

This iterative process preserves the system's integrity while accommodating growth and changing circumstances.

By applying consequences promptly, honoring every agreement, documenting rules, praising compliance, and fine-tuning outcomes together, you establish an environment where boundaries are reliable guides rather than arbitrary punishments. This consistency builds trust, models accountability, and fosters the very self-regulation you hope to instill in your adolescent. In the next chapter, we'll explore strategies for navigating those moments when even consistent consequences are challenged—equipping you with de-escalation tools and repair techniques to maintain connection under stress.

Chapter 6: When Boundaries Are Challenged

Conflict between parents and teens is as inevitable as it is challenging. As adolescents push against established limits in their quest for independence, parents often find their carefully laid boundaries under siege. Yet conflict need not be a battleground that leaves everyone wounded. In fact, when managed skillfully, these high-tension moments can become priceless opportunities for growth, understanding, and strengthened connection. This chapter—"When Boundaries Are Challenged"—is devoted to transforming the flashpoints of anger and frustration into gateways for mutual respect and deeper bonding.

We begin by demystifying the anatomy of a family dispute. Recognizing that heightened emotions can hijack even the best intentions, we'll explore practical de-escalation techniques designed to keep both voices—and hearts—steady. By learning to speak calmly, listen reflectively, and offer limited choices rather than ultimatums, parents and teens alike can shift from defensiveness to dialogue. These tools don't just defuse individual conflicts; they build an atmosphere of safety, letting each person feel heard and valued even in disagreement.

But sometimes, no matter how prepared you are, the heat of the moment demands a strategic pause. That's where carefully crafted "time-outs" come in—not as punishments, but as respectful intermissions. You'll discover how to set up neutral signals, agree on time limits, and choose personal retreat spots that allow both teen and parent to cool off without feeling abandoned or shamed. Importantly, this isn't a digital detox zone; screens and distractions are set aside in favor of mindful breathing, journaling, or other calming practices that foster genuine emotional reset.

Equally crucial is what happens once emotions have settled. Unresolved tension can breed resentment, undermining trust just when you need it most. We'll guide you step by step through the repair process: how to initiate a caring check-in, offer heartfelt apologies without caveats, and jointly devise fair compromises. By consciously expressing appreciation and planning positive shared activities—whether cooking dinner together or taking a walk—you reaffirm the core truth: your relationship transcends any single disagreement.

Ultimately, this chapter reframes conflict not as evidence of failure, but as an unavoidable—and potentially transformational— aspect of family life. When boundaries are challenged, you'll have at your fingertips a roadmap for de-escalation, a framework for restorative pauses, and a blueprint for healing afterward. These practices pave the way for healthier interactions today and lay a foundation of resilience, empathy, and mutual respect that will continue to serve your family through the turbulent teen years and well beyond.

De-escalation techniques for high-conflict moments

When tensions rise and emotions flare, a minor disagreement can quickly spiral into a full-blown argument that leaves both parent and teen feeling unheard, frustrated, and distant. Mastering de-escalation isn't about "winning" the exchange—it's about keeping lines of communication open, preserving safety, and guiding both parties back toward calm and collaboration. The techniques below form a toolkit you can draw on whenever you feel a conflict intensifying.

Regulate Your Own State First

Why it matters: Emotional contagion is real—your stress, anger, or anxiety can feed your teen's. By intentionally calming yourself first, you model composure and reduce the odds of a shouting match.

- **Pause and breathe.** Before responding, take three slow, deliberate breaths. Focus on the rise and fall of your chest.

- **Notice physical cues.** Tensing shoulders, clenched jaw, pounding heart—these are your "red light" signals to slow down.

- **Use a grounding technique.** Name five things you can see, four you can touch, three you can hear, two you can smell, and one you can taste. This sensory check-in brings your nervous system down a notch.

Speak with a Calming Tone and Open Body Language

Why it matters: Our nonverbal signals carry far more weight than words alone. A soft voice and relaxed posture communicate safety and respect.

- **Lower, even pace.** Consciously reduce your speaking volume—an immediate cue that the environment is shifting from "battle" to "conversation."

- **Open posture.** Keep arms uncrossed, shoulders relaxed, and knees slightly bent rather than locked. If possible, sit at the same level as your teen rather than looming over them.

- **Maintain comfortable eye contact.** Too little eye contact can feel dismissive; too much can feel confrontational. Aim for a soft, intermittent gaze.

Reflective ("Active") Listening

Why it matters: Teens often just want to be heard. Reflective listening signals genuine attention and helps clarify misunderstandings before they escalate.

- **Invite them to speak.** "I want to understand your perspective —tell me what's on your mind."

- **Listen fully.** Don't interrupt or rehearse your rebuttal.

- **Paraphrase and validate.** "So you felt hurt when I…" or "It sounds like you're frustrated because…"

- **Ask clarifying questions.** "When you say you felt ignored, what did that look like?"

This simple cycle—Invite → Listen → Paraphrase → Clarify— can transform a tense monologue into a cooperative dialogue.

Use "I" Statements to Express Needs

Why it matters: Framing your concerns around your own feelings prevents teens from tuning out or jumping into a defensive stance.

- **Structure:** "I feel [emotion] when [behavior or situation], because [impact]. In the future, I need [specific request]."

- **Example:** "I feel worried when chores aren't done because I'm concerned about how you manage responsibilities. In the future, I need you to finish your chores before screen time."

By owning the feeling ("I feel worried") rather than attributing blame ("You're lazy"), you invite collaboration rather than opposition.

Offer Limited, Structured Choices

Why it matters: Conflict often arises from a teen's need for autonomy bumping against a parent's need for rules. Offering choices restores a sense of control without sacrificing necessary boundaries.

- **Define the non-negotiable.** Identify the limit that cannot be crossed (e.g., homework must be completed by 7 pm).

- **Offer two acceptable options.** "You can work on your homework at the kitchen table, or in your room with the door open."

- **Follow through respectfully.** Once a choice is made, honor it. This builds trust in the process.

Establish a "Cooling Threshold" Agreement

Why it matters: Agreeing ahead of time on what constitutes an escalation worthy of a pause removes ambiguity in the moment.

- **Choose a signal.** Could be raising a hand, ringing a small bell, or saying "timeout."

- **Set parameters.** "If either of us raises our voice above a normal speaking volume three times, or we go in circles on the same point twice, we call a time-out."

- **Define the break.** A five- to ten-minute pause with clear re-entry guidelines ("We'll check in at the timer's end").

Having this agreement in place beforehand means neither side feels ambushed or infantilized when a pause is called.

Use Gentle Humor or a Shared Ritual

Why it matters: Humor—used sensitively—can break tension by shifting focus. Shared rituals remind both parties of underlying connection.

- **Humorous self-deprecation.** If you've forgotten something trivial ("Okay, apparently my brain is on vacation today!"), it can diffuse irritation.

- **Light-hearted check-ins.** A "fist bump" or quick "sorry dance" before restarting signals that you're on the same team.

- **Agree on a funny code word** for minor mishaps. Laughing together over "pineapple" instead of escalating demonstrates resilience.

Transition to Problem-Solving

Why it matters: Once emotional temperature has dropped, moving toward cooperative solutions cements the de-escalation.

- **Agree on the issue.** "It seems like the core problem is…"

- **Brainstorm jointly.** Generate options without critique: "What could work?"

- **Select and commit.** Choose the best idea and set a clear plan.

- **Schedule a follow-up.** Decide when to check on how the solution is going—tomorrow evening, for example.

De-escalation is both an art and a practice. By regulating your own state, communicating with calm clarity, listening reflectively, offering structured choices, and having transparent pause arrangements, you build a resilient framework for even the most charged disagreements. Over time, these techniques become second nature—transforming high-conflict moments into stepping stones for deeper understanding and trust.

Safe spaces and time-outs—for parent and teen

Creating designated "safe spaces" and agreed-upon time-outs transforms emotional flashpoints into intentional pauses—

moments to regroup rather than erupt. When implemented thoughtfully, these tools teach both parents and teens how to self-regulate, respect each other's needs, and return to the conversation ready to engage constructively. Below is a detailed roadmap for establishing and using safe spaces and time-outs effectively.

The Purpose and Benefits

Emotional Regulation

- Time-outs interrupt the fight-or-flight cycle, giving both parties the chance to calm down physiologically and mentally.

- Safe spaces cue the brain that it's okay to step back, breathe, and gain perspective.

Respecting Autonomy

- Teens learn that they have agency over their emotional state and environment.

- Parents model that it's healthy and responsible to acknowledge when emotions need tending.

Preventing Power Struggles

- A formalized pause removes the "winner/loser" dynamic that often fuels conflict.

- It reframes observation—"I need a break"—as a collaborative strategy rather than avoidance.

Designing Your Safe Spaces

A "safe space" is simply a chosen spot where someone can retreat to reset emotionally. It doesn't have to be elaborate—what matters is that both parent and teen respect each other's choices and boundaries.

For Teens

Let Them Choose

- Empower your teen to pick a spot that feels comforting: a cozy chair, a bean-bag, a little reading nook, or even a blanket fort.

Stock It Appropriately

- Include a few calming tools: a stress ball, sketchpad and pencils, a favorite book, or a small journal.

Personalize and Protect

- Signs like "Do Not Disturb" can signal to others that they're in their reset zone.

- Make clear that this space is a judgment-free zone; they won't be tracked down there for additional chores or demands.

For Parents

Identify Your Retreat

- It might be as simple as stepping onto a balcony, heading to a home office, or settling with a cup of tea in the kitchen.

Equip Your Space

- Keep a small "toolbox" of soothing items: headphones for quiet music or guided meditation, a few index cards with positive affirmations, or a mindfulness app on your phone.

Set Clear Boundaries

- Let family members know this is your emotional reset corner. A simple sign or a closed-door policy works.

Establishing the Time-Out Agreement

A time-out works best when everyone understands the rules *before* emotions run high.

Negotiate Calmly, Ahead of Time

- During a neutral moment, discuss why time-outs can help and co-create the guidelines.

Define the Trigger

- Examples: raised voices, repeated interruptions, walking away and slamming doors, or simply saying "I need a break."

Set the Duration

- Five to fifteen minutes is usually sufficient for heart rates to slow and thinking to clear.

- Use a timer or phone alarm; avoid clock-watching.

Agree on Re-Entry Signals

- Decide how you'll signal readiness to resume: a gentle knock, a verbal "I'm ready," or removing a "time-out" card from the door.

Clarify Non-Negotiables

- Make clear that safety (physical or emotional) always overrides the time-out—if something is urgent, the space must open.

Protocol for Taking a Time-Out

When tension builds:

Invoke the Signal

- Calmly use the agreed cue: "Time-out," raise your hand, or place the designated card on the table.

Withdraw to Your Space

- Each person goes to their chosen safe space. No trailing behind or attempts to continue the argument.

Engage in Calming Activities

- Encourage breathing exercises, gentle stretches, journaling, or listening to a soothing playlist.

- Screen time is discouraged; the goal is emotional reconnection, not distraction.

Check Physical and Mental State

- After a few minutes, rate calmness on a simple scale (1–5). If below 3, continue the break.

Re-Engaging After Time-Out

The return to conversation is as critical as the break itself.

Use a Neutral Opener

- "I'm ready to talk now. How are you feeling?"

Share Reset Reflections

- Each person briefly describes what helped them calm down and any lingering feelings: "I felt calmer after deep breathing but still a bit upset about…"

Reaffirm Mutual Respect

- "Thank you for giving me space—I want us to find a solution together."

Shift to Problem-Solving

- Review the core issue succinctly and brainstorm next steps. Aim for at least two options before deciding on one.

Troubleshooting Common Challenges

One Person Refuses the Break

- Revisit the pre-agreed rules. If necessary, enlist a trusted third party (another adult) to mediate the initial discussion.

Time-Out Becomes Avoidance

- If one party repeatedly refuses to re-engage, schedule a formal check-in later that day to process emotions and revisit the solution.

Safe Space Violations

- If someone enters another's safe zone during a time-out, pause the process and renegotiate boundaries immediately afterward.

Safe spaces and time-outs are not about punishment or avoidance; they're deliberate practices that honor each person's emotional experience. By jointly designing spaces, agreeing on clear triggers and durations, and committing to respectful re-engagement, families can transform potential blow-ups into structured, healing pauses—fostering resilience, empathy, and stronger bonds that endure well beyond the moment of conflict.

Repairing the relationship post-conflict

After the heat of an argument has cooled, emotional residue often lingers. Unspoken hurts, lingering resentment, or uncertainty about how to move forward can undermine the gains made by de-escalation and time-outs. Repair work is the bridge that reunites parent and teen, restoring trust and demonstrating that disagreements—even intense ones—can strengthen rather than fracture a relationship. Below is a detailed, step-by-step framework for repairing the bond after conflict.

Initiate a Caring Check-In

Timing and Tone

- **Within 24 Hours.** Aim to reconnect before the day ends, once both parties have had space to process.

- **Neutral Setting.** Choose a relaxed context—over a cup of tea, during a short walk, or while folding laundry.

- **Open Invitation.** Begin with a simple, low-pressure prompt: "Hey, can we check in? I've been thinking about our conversation and want to know how you're feeling."

Key Elements

Express Continued Concern

- "I still care about how you're doing after our disagreement."

Invite Their Voice

- "What's on your mind right now?"

Listen Without Defensiveness

- Make eye contact, nod, and refrain from interrupting—even if it feels critical.

Offer and Accept Sincere Apologies

An apology isn't a sign of weakness; it's a testament to respect and accountability. In families, modeling genuine remorse teaches teens how to own mistakes and make amends.

Crafting an Effective Apology

- **Be Specific.** Name the action: "I'm sorry I snapped at you…"

- **Acknowledge Impact.** Show empathy: "…and I realize that hurt your feelings."

- **Avoid Excuses.** Skip "but…" or "if…" statements that undercut sincerity.

- **Commit to Change.** Suggest a concrete step: "…next time I'll pause and breathe before responding."

Receiving an Apology

- **Accept Gracefully.** "Thank you for saying that; I appreciate it."

- **Express Your Feelings.** "It means a lot to me that you recognize how I felt."

- **Offer Reciprocity.** If you owe an apology, follow the same principles.

Collaborate on Fair Solutions

Reaching a shared solution cements repair by focusing on mutual needs and responsibilities.

Define the Core Issue

- Summarize neutrally: "So the main problem was that chores weren't finished before screen time."

Brainstorm Together

- Encourage creativity: "What ideas do you have to make this work?"

- List every suggestion without judgment.

Evaluate Options

- Discuss pros and cons: "Doing 30 minutes of homework first gives you free time later, but you might feel rushed."

Agree on a Plan

- Set clear steps: who does what, by when, and how you'll check in.

- Example: "Let's agree you'll start homework by 5:30 pm, and I'll check in at 6:15."

Document the Agreement

- Write it on a whiteboard or in a shared journal, so both can refer back.

- Seeing it in writing reinforces commitment.

Express Genuine Appreciation

Gratitude turns focus from past wounds to the strengths of your relationship. It signals to each other that respect and care prevail over conflict.

Highlight Specific Efforts

- "I appreciate how you listened during our check-in."

- "Thank you for choosing to come back and talk rather than storming off."

Acknowledge Growth

- "I've noticed you've been more proactive about homework all week."

Encourage Continued Positives

- "It really helped me see that we can work through tough stuff together."

Plan a Positive Shared Activity

Shared enjoyable experiences reinforce connection and create new, positive memories to outweigh negative ones.

Choosing the Right Activity

• **Low Pressure.** Something neither side can "lose" at, like cooking, walking, or building a simple puzzle.

• **Mutual Interest.** Ideally, both parent and teen find it engaging. Rotate choices to ensure fairness.

Structuring the Time

• **Set Aside Uninterrupted Time.** Block 30–60 minutes without screens or chores.

• **Mindful Presence.** Agree to stay focused on the activity and each other.

• **Reflect Briefly.** Afterward, share one thing each of you enjoyed about the time together.

Integrate Repair into Routine Check-Ins

Repair shouldn't be a one-off event but the start of an ongoing practice of connection.

• **Weekly Family Meeting.** Fifteen minutes to share highs, lows, and any small conflicts needing attention.

• **Emotion Check Cards.** Keep a set of cards with faces or words (e.g., "stressed," "happy") to help teens articulate feelings.

• **"Safe Word" for Check-Backs.** Agree on a phrase ("Can we circle back?") that signals a desire to revisit a topic calmly.

Learn and Adapt

Every conflict and repair cycle offers lessons for the future. Debriefing enhances resilience and understanding.

- **Reflect Individually.** Each person considers: What helped? What could go better next time?

- **Share Insights.** In a calm moment, exchange one or two reflections.

- **Adjust Agreements.** Update your time-out rules, solution strategies, or appreciation practices as needed.

Repairing the relationship post-conflict is where true resilience and empathy are forged. By initiating caring check-ins, offering heartfelt apologies, co-creating fair solutions, and weaving appreciation and positive activities into your routine, families transform painful moments into opportunities for deepened trust. Over time, this intentional repair practice becomes a hallmark of your family culture — one where disagreements are not derailments but invitations to grow closer, together.

Part III: Bridges

Part III: Bridges shifts the focus from enforcing limits to rebuilding connection. Once safety and respect are reestablished through clear boundaries, it's time to cultivate empathy and open lines of communication. These chapters introduce techniques for truly listening to your teen's experience—reflective listening, validation, and "repair talk" scripts that help both of you express needs without triggering defensiveness. By approaching difficult conversations with genuine curiosity rather than judgment, you begin to mend the emotional rifts that underlie abusive behavior.

Building bridges also means moving from a top-down model of authority to one of collaboration. In Part III, you'll learn how to co-create solutions with your adolescent, giving them real agency in problem-solving while you guide the process. Family meetings, joint goal-setting exercises, and shared decision protocols transform rules into agreements you both own. This collaboration fosters accountability and teaches vital life skills—negotiation, compromise, and creative conflict resolution—that will serve your teen well beyond the family arena.

Finally, Part III expands the support network beyond the parent–child dyad. We'll explore when and how to bring in professional resources—therapists, support groups, school counselors—and leverage community programs that reinforce the work you're doing at home. Whether it's enrolling in a family therapy group or connecting your teen with a peer-led workshop on emotional regulation, external support serves as a vital reinforcement. By weaving these bridges—empathic dialogue, joint problem-solving, and broader support—you create a comprehensive path toward lasting healing and reconnection.

Chapter 7: Rebuilding Connection Through Empathy

Conflict—even when handled respectfully—can leave an emotional residue that makes genuine connection feel out of reach. Empathy is the bridge that spans that gap, inviting both parent and teen to step into one another's inner world, understand each other's experience, and co-create a sense of safety and belonging. In this chapter, we'll explore how empathy becomes the cornerstone of healing: first by tuning in through active listening and validating feelings; next by adopting reflective rather than reactive responses; and finally by engaging in structured repair talk ("I feel… when you… because…") that transforms blame into understanding.

Empathy begins with the willingness to listen—not just to words, but to the unspoken currents of emotion beneath them. Active listening invites teens to share honestly, knowing their feelings will be met with genuine curiosity rather than judgment. As parents mirror back what they hear, and label the emotions they sense, teens gain the experience of being truly seen. This validation doesn't mean agreement; it simply says, "Your feelings matter to me." Over time, this practice rewires the family dynamic from one of negotiation and correction to one of heartfelt exchange.

But listening alone isn't enough. In the heat of a charged moment or in the aftermath of a disagreement, parents and teens alike can slip into knee-jerk, reactive patterns—conflict reflexes that replay old power dynamics or unmet needs. Reflective responses, by contrast, create a pause: a moment in which you choose understanding over reaction. By asking clarifying questions, acknowledging impacts, and articulating your own feelings calmly, you model emotional regulation and invite reciprocity. This shifts the interaction from a tug-of-war into a collaborative search for meaning.

Finally, empathy finds its full expression in repair talk. The formula "I feel... when you... because..." gives both parties a clear, non-accusatory framework to take ownership of their feelings and actions. When parents say, "I feel worried when you come home late because I fear for your safety," they open a door for teens to express their own perspective without feeling cornered. Likewise, teens can mirror that structure to communicate hurt or disappointment, upgrading complaints into invitations for change.

Throughout these three interconnected practices—active listening with validation, reflective rather than reactive responses, and structured repair talk—you'll discover that empathy isn't a passive emotion but an active skill. It requires attention, intention, and sometimes courage to name feelings both yours and theirs. Yet as you practice, you'll witness conflict moments transform into opportunities for deeper understanding, greater trust, and a parent-teen bond that thrives not in spite of disagreements, but because of them.

Active listening and validating feelings

Active listening is more than a courteous nod or the occasional "uh-huh." It is a deliberate, sustained practice that communicates to your teen, "I see you. I hear you. Your feelings matter." In high-conflict or emotionally charged situations, active listening serves three critical functions: it soothes heightened emotions, clarifies misunderstandings, and lays the groundwork for genuine empathy. Below is a step-by-step guide to implementing active listening with validating reflection.

Setting the Stage

Before launching into deep listening, create an environment conducive to open sharing. Ensure minimal distractions: put phones away, turn off the TV, and choose a comfortable seating arrangement where both parent and teen are at eye level. This non-verbal groundwork signals, "I'm fully present."

Invitation to Share

Begin with an open invitation that invites vulnerability without pressure. Phrases like "I'd really like to understand how you're feeling about this" or "Can you help me see what's going on for you?" establish a collaborative tone. Crucially, avoid ultimatums or corrective language in the invitation—this is a moment for listening, not lecturing.

Fully Receive the Message

Once your teen begins to speak, practice the art of "quiet presence."

- **Physical cues**: Lean slightly forward, uncross arms, relax your facial muscles.

- **Verbal encouragers**: Use minimal responses—"I see," "Go on," or a gentle "Tell me more."

- **Resist the urge** to plan your response or interrupt. Instead, treat each pause as an opportunity to stay with their experience.

Reflect and Label

After your teen shares a thought or feeling, mirror back what you've heard. Reflection can follow the pattern: "It sounds like you're feeling [emotion] because [situation]." For example:

"It sounds like you're feeling overwhelmed because you've got back-to-back assignments and no break."

Labeling the emotion ("overwhelmed") serves two functions: it reassures your teen that you're attuned to their inner state, and it helps them develop emotional vocabulary.

Validate Without Condoning

Validation is not agreement; it's acknowledgment of legitimacy. Phrases such as "I understand why you'd feel that way" or "I can see how that would be really frustrating" communicate respect. By validating, you're saying, "Your feelings make sense, even if the situation is challenging." This dramatically reduces defensiveness and opens the door to collaborative problem-solving.

Clarify Through Open-Ended Questions

Once you've reflected and validated, gently probe for deeper understanding:

- "What was the hardest part about that day?"

- "How did you handle it in the moment?"

- "What did you wish had been different?"
  These questions deepen the conversation, uncovering underlying concerns that might otherwise simmer unnoticed.

Check for Accuracy

End your listening cycle by asking, "Did I get that right? Is there anything I missed?" This final step ensures you haven't misunderstood or oversimplified their experience.

Transition Thoughtfully

After the active-listening loop, you can move toward problem-solving or supportive feedback. Preface this shift: "Thank you for sharing that—how can I support you now?" This reinforces that the next steps are cooperative, not corrective.

By consistently practicing these active listening moves—invitation, presence, reflection, validation, clarification, and accuracy checking—you cultivate a home environment where teens feel safe to express even difficult emotions. Over time, this routine rewiring of communication patterns strengthens trust and reduces the frequency and intensity of future conflicts.

Reflective rather than reactive responses

In emotionally charged moments, our instinctive reactions often exacerbate conflict. A raised voice begets a raised voice; a harsh retort fuels defensiveness. Reflective responding interrupts this escalation by inserting a brief pause between stimulus and reaction—shifting from instinct to intention. Below is a framework for making reflective responses your default in interactions with your teen.

Recognize Your Emotional Triggers

Self-awareness is the cornerstone of reflective practice. Begin by mapping out the specific words, tones, or gestures that consistently trigger strong emotions in you—anger, fear, or shame. Keep a brief journal for a week, noting each time you felt "flooded" with emotion: what happened, what you felt physically, and how you reacted. This audit reveals patterns and pinpoints the "hot buttons" to watch for.

Mindful Pause Technique

When you sense a trigger—heart racing, jaw clenching—initiate a "mindful pause." This can be as simple as taking a single deep inhalation, counting silently to three, or making a brief physical gesture like touching your thumb to your forefinger. This pause disrupts the automatic reaction loop, giving your prefrontal cortex a moment to engage.

Acknowledgment of Inner State

Use the pause to internally acknowledge your emotion in neutral terms: "I notice I'm feeling angry." Naming the feeling diminishes its unconscious power and creates space to choose a response rather than react unconsciously.

Use Reflective Language

Once paused, frame your reply to foster connection rather than conflict. Reflective language follows three steps:

- **Own your feeling**: "I'm feeling upset…"

- **State observation** (fact-based): "…when I see your chores aren't done after I reminded you…"

- **Invite dialogue**: "…and I'd like to understand what happened."

Example:

"I'm feeling disappointed when the dishes aren't done after dinner, and I'd like to know what got in the way."

This structure avoids blame and opens the door for your teen to share context rather than dig in defensively.

Replace "But" with "And"

In reflective responses, avoid "but," which negates preceding empathy. Instead, use "and" to connect acknowledgment and expectation:

- Reactive: "I get you're tired, but you still have to do your homework."

- Reflective: "I understand you're tired, and you still need to finish your homework before screen time."

Ask Curiosity-Driven Questions

Instead of rhetorical or leading questions, opt for genuine curiosity:

- "What part of the assignment do you find most challenging?"

- "How could we adjust your schedule so you have enough downtime?"

These questions shift the dynamic from power struggle to partnership.

Model Vulnerability

Transparency about your own emotional work encourages reciprocity. You might say, "I'm working on staying calm when I'm stressed about bills, so if I sound snappy, please remind me." This levels the playing field and normalizes emotional regulation as a shared family skill.

Follow Through with Clear Next Steps

After the reflective exchange, collaboratively decide on concrete actions. For example: "Let's agree that I'll remind you once, then you'll use a checklist to track chores." Documenting these steps reinforces accountability and reduces future ambiguity.

By embedding these reflective techniques into daily interactions, you transform potential conflicts into opportunities to model emotional intelligence. Your teen learns that emotions can be named, felt, and navigated without derailing communication or trust.

Repair talk: "I feel… when you… because…"

Repair talk crystallizes empathy into a clear, three-part framework that promotes accountability and solutions over blame. By structuring difficult conversations around personal feeling, observed behavior, and impact, both parent and teen can express themselves honestly while minimizing defensiveness. Below is a comprehensive guide to utilizing this formula effectively.

Choose the Right Moment

Repair talk is most effective when emotions have settled but the issue remains salient. Aim for a calm window—later the same day or the next—in a neutral setting free of distractions. Avoid initiating repair immediately after a heated exchange when residual adrenaline may still distort perceptions.

Introduce the Structure

Explain the reason for using this approach:

"I'd like us to try a clear way of talking about what happened so we both feel heard and can move forward."

Naming the structure upfront sets expectations and reduces resistance to the form.

Component 1: "I feel..."

Begin by naming your emotion. Using emotional vocabulary beyond the usual "upset" deepens understanding. Examples include: anxious, disappointed, overlooked, relieved, worried, or proud. Specificity builds trust:

"I feel anxious..."

Component 2: "...when you..."

Describe the concrete behavior or event. Stick to observable actions without interpretation. Avoid words like "always" or "never"—they exaggerate and trigger defensiveness. For example:

"...when you left the house without telling me..."

Component 3: "...because..."

Explain the personal impact of the behavior: the fear, inconvenience, or unmet expectation that resulted. This connects actions to emotions in a transparent way. For example:

"…because I didn't know if you were safe and I was worried you might have missed your bus."

Putting it all together:

"I feel anxious when you leave the house without telling me because I don't know if you're safe."

Inviting the Teen's Perspective

After speaking, pause and invite your teen to share theirs using the same formula. For instance:

"Can you share how you felt when I asked you to text me before you left?"

This reciprocity balances the exchange and ensures mutual understanding.

Crafting Forward-Looking Requests

Immediately following repair statements, make a clear request for future behavior:

"…so could you let me know when you're heading out next time?"

Requests should be specific, achievable, and positively framed.

Responding to Your Teen's Repair Talk

When your teen uses the formula:

- **Acknowledge their feeling**: "I hear that you felt embarrassed…"
- **Thank them**: "Thank you for telling me that."

- **Validate**: "I understand why it felt that way."

- **Commit**: "I'll do my best to ask before giving you suggestions next time."

This mirrors the empathy and accountability you modeled.

Documenting Agreements

After both parties have spoken and made requests, jot down key points on a shared medium—a whiteboard, a notes app, or a sticky note. Seeing it in writing cements the commitment and serves as a gentle reminder.

Reinforcement Through Follow-Up

Schedule a brief check-in (later that day or the next) to review how well the new agreement is working. Use the repair formula again if needed to fine-tune the arrangement.

By integrating repair talk into your conflict resolution toolkit, you foster a family culture where mistakes become opportunities for growth, rather than sources of resentment. The simple "I feel... when you... because..." template empowers both parent and teen to express honest emotions, take responsibility for actions, and collaboratively build a foundation of renewed trust and understanding.

Chapter 8: Collaborative Problem-Solving

Conflict often arises when parents and teens feel locked in opposing camps—rules versus freedom, safety versus autonomy. Collaborative problem-solving breaks down this binary by inviting both sides to pool their perspectives, needs, and creativity. Rather than parents unilaterally dictating solutions or teens resisting every boundary, this approach positions the family as a team tackling a shared challenge. In this chapter, we'll begin with a look at why co-creating solutions with your teen fosters ownership, motivation, and mutual respect. You'll see how shifting from "my way or the highway" to "let's figure this out together" sets the stage for lasting cooperation.

Next, we'll dive into practical negotiation skills and cultivate a win-win mindset. True negotiation isn't about haggling for advantage; it's about uncovering underlying interests and crafting agreements where everyone's core needs are met. We'll cover how to identify non-negotiables, brainstorm creative options, and use neutral criteria—rather than power or persuasion—to land on solutions your teen feels invested in.

Finally, we'll explore how to set up family meetings that actually work. Too often, "family meetings" become gripe sessions or one-sided lectures. We'll share a clear agenda structure, timing guidelines, and facilitation tips that keep discussions focused, respectful, and productive. You'll learn how to rotate leadership roles so teens gain experience guiding conversations, how to track agreements with simple visual tools, and how to follow up in ways that reinforce accountability without micromanagement.

By the end of this chapter, you'll have a comprehensive toolkit for transforming recurring conflicts into collaborative projects.

Whether it's curfew times, screen usage, or division of chores, you'll know how to engage your teen's voice, negotiate with empathy, and maintain momentum through effective family meetings. Collaborative problem-solving nurtures not just immediate solutions but essential life skills: communication, creativity, and compromise. As you apply these practices, you'll see your family dynamic evolve into one where challenges become opportunities for connection and growth—together.

Co-creating solutions: giving your teen agency

Granting teens a genuine role in shaping solutions does more than smooth over one-off conflicts; it builds their sense of competence and responsibility for the long haul. When teens feel they've contributed meaningfully to a rule or routine, they're far more likely to follow through—and to collaborate on future challenges. Below is a step-by-step guide to co-creating solutions that honor both parental concerns and teen autonomy.

Frame the Issue as a Shared Challenge

Begin by defining the problem neutrally—avoid "you always" or "you never." For example: "We keep bumping heads over your evening screen time and homework balance. How can we solve this so you feel you have downtime but also get your work done?" This framing conveys partnership: "us versus task," not "parent versus teen."

Identify Underlying Needs

Invite each person to articulate what matters most. Parents might say: "I need to know you're managing your responsibilities so you don't fall behind." Teens might say: "I need time to unwind and catch up with friends or creative projects." Acknowledge each need as valid. Writing them on a whiteboard or note-taking app keeps them visible and prevents reversion to positions.

Brainstorm without Judgment

Set a rule: no idea is too wild in the brainstorming phase. Encourage both sides to generate as many options as possible—timers, shared calendars, block schedules, negotiated tech-free windows, work-first incentives, or screen-time tokens. Quantity breeds creativity; aim for at least ten ideas.

Evaluate Options Collaboratively

Review the brainstormed list together, discussing pros and cons of each idea in relation to the needs identified. Use neutral criteria such as feasibility, fairness, and alignment with family values. For example: "This option gives you four hours of downtime but might push your bedtime too late—can we tweak it?" This evaluation shifts the focus away from personal gain toward objective solution-finding.

Select and Refine a Solution

Agree on one or two options to pilot. Define specifics: who does what, by when, and how success will be measured. For instance: "Let's try a 'homework first' rule: you start school tasks by 5:30 pm; once they're done, you earn up to 90 minutes of screen time. We'll check how it's working in a week." Document these details clearly—on a shared digital note or family calendar.

Set a Review Date

Agency includes accountability. Schedule a brief check-in (in person or via message) at the agreed-upon time. Questions to guide the review: "Did the plan meet both your need for downtime and my need for school progress?" "What's working well? What needs tweaking?" This follow-up completes the co-creation cycle and ensures continuous improvement.

Celebrate Successes

When the solution works, acknowledge it. A simple "I'm proud of how you managed your time this week" reinforces positive behavior and underscores the collaborative spirit. If adjustments are needed, treat them as a joint problem-solving opportunity rather than a regression.

By involving your teen from problem definition through evaluation and review, you cultivate their decision-making muscles. They learn that adult guidance and teen perspective both have value—that rules crafted together feel fairer and stick better. Over time, co-creation becomes less about conflict management and more about routine family governance that everyone helps shape.

Negotiation skills and win-win mindsets

Negotiation is often portrayed as competition—each side vying to extract the best deal. In family contexts, however, adversarial tactics backfire, breeding mistrust or compliance without commitment. A win-win mindset reframes negotiation as a collaborative exploration of mutual interests, leading to agreements that respect both parent and teen priorities. This section outlines key negotiation skills and attitudes to foster sustainable solutions.

Distinguish Positions from Interests

- **Positions**: The specific demands someone makes (e.g., "I want screen time until 10 pm").

- **Interests**: The underlying needs driving those demands (e.g., "I need time to unwind" or "I need to be well-rested for school").

Encourage both sides to articulate interests, then focus on satisfying them, which opens creative pathways that positions alone would block.

Prepare with Empathy

Before formal negotiation, parents should mentally rehearse from the teen's viewpoint—imagine their daily schedule, peer pressures, and emotional needs. Teens can do the same from the parent's perspective: responsibilities, safety concerns, and values. This empathy prep primes both parties to enter the discussion with mutual respect.

Use Neutral "Fair" Criteria

Instead of relying on power ("Because I said so"), anchor negotiation in objective standards:

- **Common routines**: "Other families often set screen curfews at 9 pm on school nights."

- **Expert recommendations**: "Health guidelines suggest eight hours of sleep for teens."

- **Family values**: "We've agreed that homework and family time take priority."
Referencing shared criteria legitimizes solutions and reduces perceptions of arbitrariness.

Leverage "If-Then" Tradeoffs

"If you complete your tasks early, then you can…" structures agreements as balanced exchanges. For example:

"If you get your homework done by 5 pm every weekday, then you can have an extra 30 minutes of screen time on Friday."

This clarifies linkages between effort and privilege, making responsibilities and rewards transparent.

Practice Active Concessions

Effective negotiators give ground strategically, making sure each concession is met with reciprocal movement. Parents might concede on small details—extending weekend curfew by 15 minutes—while teens agree to add a 10-minute nightly review of upcoming tasks. This rhythm of give-and-take fosters goodwill and prevents stagnation.

Maintain a Collaborative Tone

Language matters. Replace "you must" with "how can we?" and "my rules" with "our agreement." Phrases like "Let's figure out" or "What if we tried" emphasize partnership. Avoid ultimatums or zero-sum framing ("either the chores or the video game").

Document Agreements Visually

Writing negotiated terms on a shared board or digital note reinforces commitment. Use simple checklists or charts with clear deadlines and responsibilities. Visual documentation transforms abstract promises into concrete reminders that guide behavior.

Debrief and Iterate

At the next family check-in, review not only whether the agreement held, but also how the process worked: "Did our negotiation feel fair? What could we do differently next time?" This meta-conversation upgrades negotiation skills over time, building confidence and mutual trust.

By mastering these negotiation skills and consistently seeking win-win outcomes, families shift from power struggles to problem-solving collaborations. Teens learn respectful advocacy; parents model fairness and flexibility. Together, you build a culture where agreements address core interests, not surface positions—ensuring solutions endure beyond the immediate conflict.

Setting up family meetings that work

Regular family meetings can institutionalize collaborative problem-solving, offering a structured forum for addressing ongoing challenges, celebrating successes, and refining agreements. Yet without clear design, they quickly devolve into gripe sessions or lopsided lectures. Below is a blueprint for creating family meetings that are engaging, efficient, and genuinely democratic.

Establish a Consistent Schedule

- **Frequency**: Weekly or biweekly is often ideal—frequent enough to stay on top of issues, but not so often that attendance feels burdensome.

- **Duration**: Aim for 30–45 minutes. Longer meetings risk fatigue; shorter ones may feel rushed.

- **Predictability**: Hold meetings on the same day and time (e.g., Sunday evenings) so everyone can plan around them.

Rotate Leadership Roles

- **Facilitator**: Guides the agenda, keeps time, and invites participation. Rotate this role so teens gain facilitation experience and feel ownership.

- **Note-taker**: Records decisions, action items, and next meeting's agenda. Rotate this role as well.

- **Timekeeper**: Gives gentle reminders when discussions run long, ensuring balanced participation.

Use a Structured Agenda

Opening Check-In (5 minutes): Each member shares a quick "high" and "low" from their week—builds connection before problem-solving.

Review of Action Items (5–10 minutes): Briefly revisit previous agreements; celebrate successes and note any unfinished items.

New Agenda Items (15–20 minutes): Tackle one or two top issues submitted in advance (use a shared list or jar). For each item:

- State the issue neutrally.

- Discuss needs/interests.

- Brainstorm solutions.

- Agree on next steps.

Appreciations and Wrap-Up (5 minutes): Each person names something they appreciate about another member—ends on a positive note.

Set Ground Rules

One Voice at a Time: Use a "talking object" (e.g., a small ball) passed to whomever has the floor.

No Blame Zone: Focus on behaviors and solutions, not character attacks.

Be Present: Phones and screens off or in a basket; eye contact encouraged.

Encourage Equal Participation

Teens often defer to parents. Use prompts like "What do you think?" or "Can you share another idea?" If someone is quieter, the facilitator can gently invite their input: "Alex, would you like to add anything?"

Visual Tracking of Agreements

Action Board or App: Display tasks, deadlines, and responsible parties.

Check-Off System: Provide markers for completed items—satisfying visuals reinforce progress.

Color Coding: (Optional) Different colors for chores, academics, and social plans helps categorization.

Follow-Up Between Meetings

Brief Midweek Touch-Point: A 5-minute check-in over dinner or message ensures that tasks are on track and minor tweaks can be made before next meeting.

Celebrate Milestones: Acknowledge when a new system or agreement has worked well—builds momentum.

Iterate the Process

Solicit feedback on the meeting itself: "What went well? What could we change?" Adjust agenda timing, roles, or ground rules based on the family's evolving needs.

Well-run family meetings reinforce that everyone's perspective matters and that solutions are reached through respectful dialogue. As teens take on leadership roles and see their ideas shape family life, they develop confidence, responsibility, and a sense of belonging. Parents model organization, fairness, and responsiveness. Together, you create a living governance system that adapts to new challenges and strengthens your collaborative problem-solving muscle for years to come.

Chapter 9: Therapeutic and Community Supports

Conflict and stress within parent–teen relationships can sometimes exceed what family strategies alone can resolve. Recognizing when additional expertise or peer support is needed is not a sign of failure, but rather of commitment to health and growth. In this chapter, we explore three vital realms of help beyond the family's walls: **when to seek professional help**, **group programs**, and **school-based and community resources**. Each offers specialized tools, impartial perspectives, and structured environments that can accelerate healing, foster resilience, and equip both parents and teens with new skills.

First, we'll look at **when to seek professional help**. Therapists, social workers, and other mental-health professionals bring deep training in communication dynamics, emotional regulation, and trauma-informed care. We'll discuss common red flags that indicate it's time to call in a pro, how to find the right fit, and what to expect in individual, family, or couples-style sessions.

Next, we'll turn to **group programs**, including family therapy and teen support groups. These settings leverage the power of shared experience: teens discover they're not alone in their struggles, parents learn from one another, and the structured format of group sessions fosters accountability. You'll learn how to evaluate program curricula, decide between open-enrollment versus cohort models, and prepare for the unique dynamics of peer sharing.

Finally, we'll examine **school-based and community resources**, from on-site counseling and lunch-hour drop-in clubs to neighborhood nonprofit workshops and online forums. These accessible supports often remove barriers of cost and transportation, making early intervention more feasible. We'll map out how to navigate school policies, build partnerships with counselors and coaches, and tap into local youth-development organizations.

Together, these three sections offer a comprehensive guide to expanding your toolkit beyond the living room. Whether you're grappling with anxiety, substance-use concerns, academic burnout, or a sense of disconnection, knowing where and when to turn—and how to choose among myriad options—can make all the difference. By integrating professional expertise, peer solidarity, and community networks into your family's support system, you safeguard not only today's relationship but also your teen's long-term emotional well-being.

When to seek professional help (therapists, social workers)

Navigating adolescence can surface complex challenges—depression, anxiety, mood swings, self-harm ideation, or escalating family conflict—that exceed the scope of typical parenting strategies. Professional help fills that gap with specialized knowledge, confidentiality, and therapeutic techniques tailored to individual needs. Here's how to recognize the signs, choose the right professional, and engage effectively in therapy:

Recognizing Red Flags

Persistent Emotional Distress

Intense sadness, irritability, or anxiety lasting more than two weeks.

Frequent crying spells or tearfulness unrelated to situational triggers.

Functional Impairment

Slipping grades, school avoidance, or unexplained absences.

Withdrawal from friends, hobbies, or family activities once enjoyed.

Self-Harm or Suicidal Talk

Cutting, burning, or other self-injuring behaviors.

Expressions of hopelessness or direct talk of suicide.

Substance Misuse

Regular use of alcohol or drugs, especially to cope with stress or emotions.

Legal or disciplinary issues related to substances.

Escalating Family Tension

Chronic power struggles, yelling matches, or physical intimidation.

A breakdown in communication despite consistent home-based efforts.

If any of these patterns emerge, it's time to consult a professional. Early intervention often prevents escalation and supports healthier coping skills.

Types of Professionals

Licensed Mental Health Counselors (LMHCs) & Psychologists

Provide talk therapy (CBT, DBT, family systems work).

Often specialize in adolescent development or specific issues (eating disorders, trauma).

Psychiatrists

Medical doctors who can prescribe and manage psychiatric medications.

Work in tandem with therapists for combined therapy-medication plans.

Social Workers (LCSWs)

Offer case management, family therapy, and connections to community resources.

Skilled in navigating school systems, social services, and crisis intervention.

School Counselors

On-site advocates who address academic, social, and emotional needs.

Can provide short-term counseling and referrals to outside services.

Finding the Right Fit

Clarify Goals

Are you seeking individual support for your teen, family therapy, or parent coaching?

Prioritize professionals whose expertise aligns with your primary concern.

Insurance and Budget

Check coverage for therapy, medication management, or social-work services.

Explore sliding-scale clinics or community-based agencies if cost is an issue.

Credentials and Specialties

Verify licensure (e.g., "LPCC," "LCSW," or "PhD/PsyD").

Look for experience with adolescents and families.

Availability and Location

Consider proximity, evening/weekend hours, and telehealth options.

Test responsiveness with an initial phone consultation.

What to Expect in Therapy

Intake and Assessment

Initial sessions focus on building rapport, gathering history, and setting goals.

Therapeutic Techniques

- **Cognitive-Behavioral Therapy (CBT):** Identifies and reframes negative thought patterns.

- **Dialectical Behavior Therapy (DBT):** Teaches emotion-regulation and distress-tolerance skills.

- **Family Systems Therapy:** Examines interaction patterns and builds healthier dynamics.

Session Rhythm

Typically weekly or biweekly, 45–60 minutes each.

Progress is reviewed every 4–6 weeks, with goals adjusted as needed.

Confidentiality and Consent

Teens over a certain age can request confidentiality; discuss limits (harm to self/others).

Parents should maintain open communication about the therapeutic process while respecting teen privacy.

Maximizing Benefits

Consistent Attendance

Regular sessions build trust and momentum.

Homework and Practice

Many therapists assign exercises (journaling, skill drills) between sessions.

Parallel Parent Work

Parent-only sessions or groups help caregivers learn supportive techniques.

Integrated Care

Coordinate between school counselors, medical providers, and therapists for a unified approach.

Seeking professional help demonstrates care and proactivity. With the right match and realistic expectations, therapy and social-work services can transform distress into growth, equipping both teen and parent with lifelong tools for resilience and connection.

Group programs: family therapy, teen support groups

Beyond one-on-one therapy, **group programs** harness the power of shared experience. In family therapy, multiple members work together under professional guidance; in teen support groups, adolescents connect with peers facing similar challenges. Both formats offer unique advantages: collective problem-solving, peer validation, and cost efficiencies. Here's how to evaluate and engage in group interventions:

Benefits of Group Settings

Normalization and Validation

Teens realize they're not alone in anxiety, identity struggles, or academic pressure.

Parents find solidarity in others' parenting challenges.

Skill-Building Through Modeling

Observing peers' coping strategies or parents' negotiation techniques provides live tutorials.

Accountability and Support

Group members encourage each other's progress and hold one another to commitments.

Cost and Access

Group rates are often lower than individual therapy, making services more affordable.

Types of Group Programs

Family Therapy Groups

Led by systemic-trained therapists.

Explore communication patterns, roles, and boundaries within the family unit.

Sessions range from 6–16 weeks, often meeting weekly for 90 minutes.

Teen Support Groups

Focus on specific issues: anxiety, grief, bullying, LGBTQ+ identity, substance use.

Peer-facilitated or led by a counselor.

May be open-enrollment or closed cohorts where members start and finish together.

Psychoeducational Workshops

Shorter series (4–8 sessions) teaching concrete skills: emotion regulation, study habits, conflict resolution.

Often part of community-health initiatives or nonprofit youth programs.

Choosing the Right Program

Curriculum and Focus

Review session outlines: Are topics relevant and comprehensive?

Ensure the program balances education, discussion, and experiential exercises (role-plays, art therapy).

Group Size and Format

Smaller groups (6–8 participants) foster deeper sharing; larger ones (10–12) offer broader perspectives.

Closed cohorts build cohesion; open groups allow rolling enrollment but may limit trust-building.

Facilitator Credentials

Verify licensure and specialization in adolescent or family therapy.

Look for trainers skilled in group dynamics and crisis management.

Logistics

Evaluate location accessibility, session timing, and sliding-scale options.

Ask about childcare or parallel parent and teen offerings if schedules conflict.

Preparing for Group Participation

Set Expectations

Explain confidentiality guidelines and the value of honest sharing.

Discuss potential discomfort and the importance of respectful listening.

Define Goals

Encourage each member to identify personal objectives: "I want to manage my anger better," or "I hope to improve family communication."

Establish Ground Rules

Agree on no interrupting, nonjudgmental responses, and strict confidentiality among members.

Maximizing Group Benefits

Active Engagement

Participate fully in activities and discussions; passive attendance limits growth.

Homework and Practice

Many groups assign between-session exercises—treat these as essential complements to in-session work.

Peer Support Networks

Exchange contact information (with facilitator approval) for accountability partners.

Parent-Teen Dyads

If possible, parallel groups allow teens and parents to debrief together after sessions, reinforcing mutual insights.

Transitioning Out of the Group

Final Review

Summarize key learnings, progress toward goals, and next steps.

Ongoing Maintenance

Explore alumni or booster sessions to sustain momentum.

Integration into Home Life

Plan a family check-in to share insights and create home-based action plans based on group learnings.

Group programs combine therapeutic expertise with community solidarity, offering rich environments for learning, connection, and accountability. Whether in the structured setting of family therapy or the camaraderie of teen support groups, participants gain multifaceted support that can bolster individual growth and family resilience.

School-based and community resources

While private therapy and formal groups serve many families, **school-based and community resources** often provide accessible, low-cost, or free support—crucial for early intervention and sustained help. By tapping into these local networks, parents and teens can find a continuum of services that align with academic schedules, cultural contexts, and peer ecosystems.

School-Based Supports

Guidance Counselors and School Psychologists

Offer short-term counseling, crisis intervention, and academic planning.

Can facilitate small-group workshops on stress management or social skills.

Coordinate 504 plans or individualized education programs (IEPs) for students with special needs.

Social-Emotional Learning (SEL) Programs

Integrated into curricula; teach emotional literacy, empathy, and conflict-resolution skills.

Examples include Second Step®, PBIS (Positive Behavioral Interventions and Supports), and restorative-justice circles.

Peer Mentoring and Peer Support Clubs

Trained student mentors provide guidance and a listening ear.

Clubs focused on mental health awareness, anti-bullying, or mindfulness.

After-School Enrichment and Clubs

Extracurriculars in arts, sports, or service promote belonging and stress relief.

Some schools partner with local nonprofits to offer therapeutic art or movement programs.

Community-Based Resources

Nonprofit Youth Organizations

YMCA/YWCA, Boys & Girls Clubs, and Big Brothers Big Sisters offer mentoring, lifeskills workshops, and recreational activities.

Many run specialized teen drop-in centers or weekend support groups.

Faith-Based Groups

Churches, mosques, synagogues, and interfaith centers often provide counseling, youth groups, and parent-teen retreats.

Emphasize holistic well-being—social, spiritual, and emotional.

Local Mental Health Clinics and Charities

Community clinics may offer sliding-scale or no-cost therapy, especially in underserved areas.

Organizations like Mental Health America or NAMI (National Alliance on Mental Illness) run support groups and education programs.

Online Platforms and Hotlines

Organizations such as 7 Cups, Teen Line, and Crisis Text Line provide anonymous chat and phone support.

Virtual workshops on coping skills, resilience, and digital wellness.

Navigating Access and Partnerships

Building Relationships with School Staff

Introduce yourself to the counselor or principal; share concerns and ask about available programs.

Attend PTA meetings or parent-teacher conferences to stay informed.

Community Resource Mapping

Research local directories or use tools like 211.org to find social-service agencies.

Create a shared digital document listing contacts, services, and eligibility criteria.

Advocacy and Referral

Don't hesitate to request formal referrals from pediatricians or school nurses.

Leverage faith-based or civic networks for personal introductions to trusted providers.

Integrating Supports into Family Life

Coordinated Schedules

Align school and community program times with family routines to minimize conflicts.

Use shared calendars and reminders for appointments and group meetings.

Parent Involvement

Attend relevant workshops (e.g., parenting seminars, SEL previews) to reinforce home-school continuity.

Serve as a chaperone or volunteer to deepen engagement and trust.

Follow-Through and Feedback

After each interaction—counseling session, group meeting—debrief with your teen about what resonated.

Provide feedback to program leaders to tailor offerings for your family's needs.

Monitoring Impact and Next Steps

Track Progress

Use simple metrics: attendance consistency, mood-tracking journals, academic performance.

Adjust as Needed

If a resource isn't a good fit, pivot quickly to alternatives—better to try something new than remain stuck.

Celebrate Milestones

Acknowledge strides—improved grades, fewer conflicts, stronger friendships—to reinforce commitment.

By weaving together school-based counseling, community youth programs, and grassroots support networks, families create a safety net of resources tailored to diverse needs and budgets. This integrated approach ensures that help is not a one-time event but a sustained ecosystem surrounding both parent and teen—fostering growth, connection, and well-being that extend far beyond the home.

Part IV: Sustaining Change

Part IV: Sustaining Change focuses on the long game—making sure the strides you've taken in setting boundaries and rebuilding connection don't slip back into old patterns. It begins by establishing reliable systems for tracking progress, such as weekly check-ins, behavior logs, or simple family "temperature" gauges where everyone rates how safe and respected they feel. By regularly reviewing what's working and what's still a struggle, you keep small issues from festering and celebrate incremental wins that reinforce everyone's commitment to improvement.

Next, this section tackles relapse prevention by helping both parent and teen identify common triggers—academic stress, social conflicts, or unstructured free time—and develop clear "if–then" plans to navigate them. You'll learn how to build your teen's emotional-regulation toolkit (deep breathing, journaling, physical outlets) and introduce family rituals—shared meals, weekend check-ins, or gratitude rounds—that anchor the household in predictability and mutual support. These rituals don't just fill calendars; they cultivate a sense of belonging and shared responsibility for sustaining a respectful climate.

Finally, Sustaining Change is about paving the path toward independence. As your adolescent demonstrates consistent responsibility, you'll gradually loosen certain boundaries, replacing them with coaching conversations that focus on life skills—managing money, negotiating adult relationships, or asking for help when overwhelmed. By transferring more decision-making power to your teen in a structured way, you reinforce the lessons of accountability and empathy you've taught, setting them up to thrive as self-reliant, emotionally intelligent adults.

Chapter 10: Maintaining Momentum

Change doesn't end once the initial conflict is resolved or a new agreement is inked on the family whiteboard. True transformation requires ongoing attention, reflection, and adaptation. In this final chapter, we focus on **maintaining momentum**—the practices that keep positive shifts from slipping back into old patterns. You'll learn how systematic tracking through behavior logs and weekly check-ins sustains progress; why celebrating even the smallest victories fuels motivation and reinforces good habits; and how to recalibrate boundaries as your teen grows, ensuring that rules evolve alongside their expanding capacities and responsibilities.

Sustaining progress begins with measurement. Just as athletes record workouts to monitor gains, families benefit from documenting behaviors and check-ins. A simple behavior log—tracking completed chores, homework, screen-time adherence, or verbal tone—illuminates patterns at a glance. Weekly check-ins transform those data points into meaningful conversations: What's working? Where are the snags? This rhythm of documentation plus reflection prevents small issues from snowballing and keeps everyone accountable.

But data alone won't sustain change. Emotional reinforcement is equally vital. Celebrating small successes—finishing a chore streak, managing stress without yelling, honoring deadlines two weeks in a row—creates positive feedback loops. Recognition doesn't have to be grand: a high-five, a sticky-note praise on the bathroom mirror, or a spontaneous "I noticed and appreciate…" statement can bolster self-esteem and stunt discouragement. Consistent acknowledgment communicates, "I see your effort, and it matters."

As your teen matures, yesterday's boundaries may feel constraining, and tomorrow's expectations may seem overdue.

Adolescence is a time of rapid cognitive, emotional, and social growth; what was appropriate at 13 may be infantile at 16. Adjusting boundaries dynamically—loosening curfews, granting more tech freedom, shifting chore responsibilities—honors your teen's developmental trajectory while safeguarding safety and structure. These recalibrations are best negotiated collaboratively, building on the collaborative problem-solving skills you nurtured in Chapter 8.

Throughout this chapter, we'll provide practical templates for behavior logs, sample questions for weekly check-ins, creative celebration ideas, and a framework for boundary adjustment that balances autonomy with guidance. By weaving these practices into your family's routine, you'll transform short-term wins into lasting habits, deepen mutual trust, and equip your teen with the self-regulation and negotiation skills they'll carry into adulthood. Let's explore how to keep the momentum going, so the progress you've worked so hard to achieve continues to flourish long after this book is closed.

Tracking Progress: Behavior Logs & Weekly Check-Ins

Maintaining momentum hinges on visibility—knowing exactly where you stand so you can course-correct before small lapses become entrenched problems. Behavior logs and weekly check-ins provide that visibility, turning subjective impressions into objective data and habitually scheduled reflection. Below is a step-by-step guide to implementing these tools effectively.

Designing a Simple Behavior Log

Identify Key Behaviors

Select 3–5 critical actions or metrics to track. Examples include:

Homework completion

Chore adherence

Screen-time limits

Use of respectful tone (no yelling)

Mood check (self-rated 1–5)

Choose a Format

Digital: Spreadsheet, shared calendar, or habit-tracking app.

Analog: Paper chart on the fridge or a laminated poster with dry-erase markers.

Define Measurement Criteria

Binary: Yes/No (e.g., "Chore completed: ✓/✗").

Scaled: 1–5 for quality or effort (e.g., "Mood: 4/5").

Time-Based: Minutes/hours logged (e.g., "Screen time: 1h 15m").

Assign Responsibility

Decide who logs each entry—teen, parent, or both. Joint ownership reinforces accountability.

Keep It Visible

Place logs where the family naturally congregates (kitchen, living room). Visibility fosters consistency.

Conducting Weekly Check-Ins

Schedule Consistently

Choose a reliable time—Sunday evening after dinner or Friday afternoon before screen time.

Block 15–20 minutes; short enough to respect busy lives, long enough for depth.

Prepare Prompts

Use a standard set of questions to guide reflection:

"What went well this week?"

"What challenges did you face?"

"How did our plan support you—or not?"

"What adjustments should we make?"

Review the Log Together

Highlight trends: streaks of success, recurring dips, or surprising spikes.

Celebrate achievements and empathize with difficulties.

Set Weekly Goals

Based on the log, co-create 1–2 specific goals for the upcoming week.

Ensure goals are SMART: Specific, Measurable, Achievable, Relevant, Time-bound.

Document Action Steps

Note who will do what by when, and how it will be tracked.

Update the behavior log template if necessary (e.g., add a new metric).

End Positively

Conclude with an appreciation round: "I appreciate how you tried X this week."

Reinforce shared commitment: "Let's tackle this next week as a team."

Troubleshooting Common Pitfalls

Log Fatigue

If entries become sporadic, simplify categories or reduce frequency.

Introduce gamification: stickers for consistency or a family points system redeemable for small privileges.

Defensiveness During Check-Ins

Remind yourself and your teen that the log is nonjudgmental, a tool for insight, not blame.

Use "I" statements: "I noticed the log shows…" instead of "You didn't…"

Rigid Metrics

Life happens: vacations, illness, and holidays disrupt routines. Adjust logs temporarily rather than abandoning them.

By coupling quantitative logs with qualitative weekly discussions, families build a feedback loop that sustains progress and deepens understanding. Over time, patterns emerge—both strengths to amplify and vulnerabilities to address—keeping you ahead of potential conflicts and aligned on shared goals.

Celebrating Small Successes

Momentum thrives on positive reinforcement. Even modest wins —completing a full week of agreed tasks, choosing calm words during disagreement, or independently starting homework— deserve recognition. Celebrations signal that progress, not perfection, is the goal, and that effort itself is valued. Below are strategies to integrate celebration into your family culture.

Identify Appropriate Wins

Process-Based Achievements

Effort and consistency: days without yelling, daily journaling, or consistent log entries.

Outcome-Based Successes

Completed project ahead of time, improved grades, or meeting a step-count goal.

Behavioral Milestones

First self-initiated apology, proactive problem-solving, or handling peer conflict calmly.

Create a Celebration Toolkit

Verbal Praise

Specificity matters: "I'm proud you stuck to our homework plan every night this week."

Tangible Tokens

Stickers, smiley-face magnets, or colored bracelets—small items that mark achievement.

Privilege Boosters

Extra 10 minutes of screen time, picking a movie for family night, or choosing dessert.

Quality Time Rewards

One-on-one outings: coffee run, drive-thru ice cream, or a short walk together.

Family Rituals

Victory jingles, high-five routines, or a "celebration jar" where you deposit notes of success to read at month's end.

Embedding Celebration into Routine

Link to Check-Ins and Logs

During weekly reviews, dedicate time to highlight 2–3 successes from the log.

Daily Micro-Celebrations

Catch positive moments spontaneously: "You chose calm words just now — that deserves a mini high-five."

Streak Recognition

Acknowledge consecutive days of meeting goals: after three days, mark with a sticker; after a week, unleash a larger reward.

Public Acknowledgment

Share successes in broader family contexts: grandparents, family-group chat, or a family newsletter board.

Avoiding Comparison and Overjustification

Individualized Celebrations

Tailor rewards to each teen's interests; what delights one may bore another.

Steer Clear of Bribes

Celebrations should reinforce intrinsic motivation, not become bargaining tools. Keep rewards modest and tied to genuine achievement.

Balance with Neutral Feedback

Combine praise with reflective prompts: "Great job on chores—what felt most helpful about our new schedule?"

Sustaining Motivation Over Time

Vary Rewards

Rotate privileges and activities to maintain novelty.

Scale Celebrations

Differentiate between small, medium, and large milestones with correspondingly scaled rewards.

Invite Teen Input

Have your teen suggest celebration ideas—they'll feel more ownership and anticipation.

Linking Celebration to Growth Mindset

Emphasize Effort

Celebrate strategies and persistence ("I saw you keep trying even after it was tough").

Normalize Setbacks

When failures occur, acknowledge the effort and frame next steps: "You tried; let's tweak our approach."

By weaving celebrations into daily life, families create a positive emotional climate that reinforces desired behaviors and nurtures self-esteem. Small wins accumulate, fueling confidence and signaling that change is both possible and appreciated.

Adjusting Boundaries as Your Teen Grows

Boundaries are not static barriers but dynamic frameworks that evolve as teens mature. As cognitive abilities, emotional regulation, and social responsibilities expand, so too should the latitude and expectations you entrust your teen with. Recalibrating boundaries reinforces autonomy, prevents rebellion born of overrestriction, and maintains safety by matching limits to developmental readiness.

A. Understanding Developmental Milestones

Early Adolescence (11–13)

Concrete thinkers who benefit from clear, simple rules and consistent routines.

Boundaries focus on basic safety: bedtimes, screen limits, and supervised activities.

Middle Adolescence (14–16)

Emerging abstract reasoning and identity exploration.

Gradual extension of privileges: later curfews, unsupervised socializing, and personal project time.

Late Adolescence (17–19)

Solidifying decision-making skills and preparing for independence.

Boundaries shift toward mutual agreements, contract-style autonomy, and real-world responsibilities (jobs, driving).

Signs It's Time to Revisit Boundaries

Routine Compliance

When your teen consistently meets expectations without reminders.

Demonstrated Responsibility

Managing tasks, punctuality, and self-care with minimal oversight.

Expressed Readiness

Mature discussions about privileges; clear plans for handling new freedoms.

Peer Comparisons

Friends or older siblings have privileges your teen lacks— consider developmental fairness.

Collaborative Boundary Adjustment Process

Data-Informed Discussion

Use your behavior log and weekly check-in summaries as evidence of readiness.

Mutual Needs Assessment

Parents articulate safety concerns; teens share autonomy goals.

Brainstorm New Parameters

Examples: shifting curfew by 30 minutes, replacing parental check-ins with self-check reports, increasing weekend unsupervised hours.

Pilot Period

Trial the new boundary for 2–4 weeks with clear criteria for success.

Review and Refine

During weekly check-ins, assess what's working and adjust if needed.

Examples of Boundary Evolution

Curfew Flexibility

Early Teens: 8:30 pm on school nights.

Middle Teens: 9–9:30 pm after homework completion.

Late Teens: Event-driven curfews, negotiated per activity.

Screen-Time Management

Early Teens: Parent-set limits and locks.

Middle Teens: Earned screen-time tokens via chores.

Late Teens: Trust-based usage, with self-imposed app timers.

Social Independence

Early Teens: Group outings with known peers.

Middle Teens: One-on-one gatherings with check-ins.

Late Teens: Self-directed plans and transportation.

Balancing Autonomy with Accountability

Clear Expectations

Even as boundaries loosen, define non-negotiables: safety protocols, school responsibilities, respectful communication.

Self-Reporting Mechanisms

Apps or shared logs where teens note arrival times, study hours, or expenses.

Natural Consequences

Real-world outcomes—late arrivals reduce unsupervised privileges; missed deadlines prompt academic support, not abrupt bans.

Navigating Pushback

Empathetic Listening

Acknowledge disappointment: "I know you're eager for more freedom."

Data Dialogue

Refer to logs: "You handled the last curfew extension well; let's build on that."

Consistent Follow-Through

Honor agreements; reversals without cause undermine trust.

Preparing for Full Independence

Life-Skills Emphasis

Budgeting, cooking, time management, and self-care become part of boundary discussions.

Graduated Responsibility

Link privileges to competencies: driving eligibility tied to safe driving courses and responsible in-car behavior.

Exit Strategy

Create a "handoff plan" for college or work life: emergency protocols, check-ins, and support networks.

By attentively adjusting boundaries in concert with developmental growth, parents both honor their teen's emerging autonomy and maintain the safety net essential to healthy maturation. This dynamic boundary model equips adolescents with responsibility, builds trust, and smooths the transition to adult independence—fueling a virtuous cycle of empowerment and accountability that sustains long-term success.

Chapter 11: Preventing Relapse

Even with strong routines and positive habits in place, families can sometimes slip back into old, unhelpful patterns—raised voices, missed check-ins, or unmet commitments. Preventing relapse isn't about perfection; it's about recognizing early warning signs, reinforcing new skills, and embedding supportive rituals so that progress becomes the path of least resistance. In this chapter, we'll begin by exploring how to **identify and prepare for common triggers** that tend to derail even the most motivated families. You'll learn to spot those high-risk situations—deadline pressures, peer conflicts, hormonal shifts—and build contingency plans to navigate them smoothly.

Next, we'll delve into **building emotional regulation skills in your teen**, laying out step-by-step exercises, modeling strategies, and real-world practice scenarios. Emotional regulation isn't a one-and-done lesson; it's a lifelong capacity that grows through mindful practice, compassionate coaching, and incremental challenges. We'll cover how to teach breathing exercises, use mood meters, and scaffold cognitive techniques so your teen feels empowered to manage stress without reverting to outbursts.

Finally, we'll show you how **family rituals and routines** can serve as powerful scaffolding for safety and connection. From morning check-in questions over breakfast to a weekly "gratitude circle" before bed, these predictable moments anchor new behaviors and reinforce the values you've co-created. We'll provide templates for scheduling, ideas for making rituals feel fresh rather than rote, and tips for inviting teens to co-design family ceremonies that honor their growing independence.

By combining proactive trigger management, ongoing emotional-regulation skill building, and supportive family rituals, you'll create a self-sustaining ecosystem that guards against backsliding. Rather than relying on willpower alone—which naturally ebbs and flows—you'll harness structure, connection, and shared responsibility to keep your family on track. Let's explore how to prevent relapse by anticipating challenges, nurturing resilience in your teen, and weaving safety into your everyday rituals.

Identifying and preparing for common triggers

Even the healthiest dynamics can unravel when familiar stressors emerge. By mapping common triggers and preemptively rehearsing responses, families can navigate bumps in the road without sliding back into conflict. This section guides you through conducting a "trigger audit," developing action plans, and creating quick-response tools to head off relapse.

Mapping Your Family's Trigger Landscape

Collective Brainstorm

Schedule a neutral-tone discussion. Ask each member to list moments when they felt most stressed or reactive in the past month—homework crunches, weekend plans gone awry, money worries, or amplified sibling rivalry.

Categorize Triggers

Sort them into buckets: Time Pressure (late work submissions, morning rush), Emotional Upsets (arguments with friends, romantic drama), Environmental Shifts (vacations, daylight savings), and Physical States (hunger, tiredness).

Rate Intensity and Frequency

On a 1–5 scale, rate how strongly each trigger impacts family harmony and how often it occurs. This prioritizes which scenarios to tackle first.

Creating Trigger Response Plans

Select Top Three

Focus on triggers with high intensity and frequency (e.g., Sunday evening homework meltdown or Friday-night screen disputes).

Define Early Warning Signs

For each trigger, identify subtle cues: clenched jaw, abrupt silence, eye-rolling, or repeated "I can't." Recognizing these signals early allows for timely intervention.

Draft "If-Then" Strategies

Use conditional statements to map responses:

Time Pressure: "If it's Sunday at 6 pm and homework is undone, then we initiate a 15-minute family planning huddle to allocate quiet work zones and snack breaks."

Emotional Upset: "If someone is snappy after school, then we pause for a five-minute check-in and breathing exercise before any task discussion."

Assign Roles

Decide who triggers the plan (usually the first to notice signs) and who facilitates it. Rotating this role builds collective responsibility.

Developing Quick-Response Tools

Visual Cue Cards

Laminate small cards with each "If-Then" statement and place them in common areas or on the fridge.

Digital Alerts

Set phone alarms labeled with plan prompts ("Homework Huddle!") at key times.

Emergency Calm Kits

Assemble a box containing stress balls, coloring pages, scented hand lotion, and a list of breathing scripts—tools for on-the-spot regulation.

Rehearsal and Review

Role-Play Practice

Periodically simulate trigger scenarios in low-stakes contexts— pretend it's Sunday at 6 pm with no homework done, then run through your planning huddle.

Post-Trigger Debriefs

After an actual trigger event, hold a 5-minute "After-Action Review": What went according to plan? What tripped us up? Adjust If-Then statements as needed.

Document Learnings

Keep a shared journal or digital note of real-world examples, refinements, and insights to inform future practice.

By systematically identifying and rehearsing responses to the triggers most likely to precipitate relapse, families transform reactive chaos into proactive collaboration. Early intervention prevents minor stresses from cascading into full-blown conflicts, preserving the progress you've worked so hard to achieve.

Building Emotional Regulation Skills in Your Teen

Emotional regulation is the engine of relapse prevention: teens equipped to recognize, name, and manage their internal states are far less likely to default to explosive reactions or avoidance. This section outlines a graduated program for teaching and reinforcing regulation skills, drawing on evidence-based techniques from mindfulness, cognitive-behavioral therapy, and neuroscience-informed practice.

A. Foundational Awareness Exercises

Mood Meter Check-Ins

Introduce a simple 4-quadrant chart mapping energy (low–high) against pleasantness (unpleasant–pleasant). Each morning or evening, teens place a sticker in the quadrant that matches their mood and note a brief reason ("felt rushed," "good soccer practice").

Physical Sensation Mapping

Guide teens through a body scan: identify where stress shows up —tight shoulders, stomach knots, headache—and rate intensity. This mind-body linkage lays the groundwork for early recognition.

Teaching Calming Tools

Breathing Techniques

Box Breathing: Inhale for 4 counts, hold 4, exhale 4, hold 4. Repeat until heart rate slows.

Diaphragmatic Breathing: Place a hand on the belly, breathe so the hand rises, promoting deeper, more regulated breaths.

Grounding Practices

5-4-3-2-1 Sensory Exercise: Name five things you see, four you can touch, three you hear, two you smell, one you taste. This anchors attention in the present.

Movement Breaks: Encourage quick walks, stretching, or doubling a hallway lap to dissipate physiological arousal.

Cognitive Techniques

Thought Journaling

Teach the ABC model: note the **A**ctivating event, the **B**elief or interpretation, and the **C**onsequences (emotions/behaviors). Reviewing entries helps teens spot unhelpful thinking patterns ("All or nothing" or "catastrophizing").

Reframing Practice

Role-play turning rigid thoughts into balanced alternatives: "I failed that test" → "That test was hard, but I can improve with practice."

Problem-Solving Worksheets

Structured forms guide teens to define a problem, brainstorm solutions, weigh pros/cons, select an approach, and evaluate outcomes. This formalizes reflective rather than reactive responses.

Skill Integration and Reinforcement

Daily Skill Prompts

At predetermined times (after school, before homework), text or call teens to use a particular tool—"Try box breathing for two minutes now."

Buddy System

Pair siblings or friends to practice skills together, sharing successes and challenges.

Positive Skill Feedback

When a teen uses a tool effectively—pauses instead of snapping—acknowledge it immediately: "I noticed you stepped outside to breathe before coming in. Nice work."

Gradual Challenge and Autonomy

Stress-Point Assignments

As confidence grows, assign teens to use regulation tools during mildly stressful situations—class presentations, team practices—so they generalize skills.

Self-Monitoring Checklists

Encourage teens to rate their alertness and regulation success daily, reinforcing self-efficacy.

Teen-Led Teaching

Have them teach a new regulation exercise to a parent or sibling; teaching cements mastery.

Parental Modeling and Support

Parents should practice the same tools openly: "I'm doing box breathing because I feel stressed about bills." This normalizes regulation as a shared family skill and invites partnership.

By progressively building awareness, teaching concrete tools, and providing structured practice and feedback, you equip your teen with a robust emotional-regulation toolkit. Consistent application of these strategies significantly lowers the risk of relapse into conflict-driven patterns.

Family Rituals and Routines That Reinforce Safety

Stable rituals and routines create a predictable environment that soothes anxiety, cements bonding, and reminds every family member of shared values. When thoughtfully designed, these repeated practices become automatic safety nets—guardrails that guide behavior, foster connection, and reduce the cognitive load of constant decision-making. Here's how to build and sustain rituals that prevent relapse.

Morning and Evening Anchors

Morning "High-Low" Check

Over breakfast, each person names a "high" and "low" they anticipate for the day. This primes supportive mindsets and uncovers potential stressors early.

Evening Gratitude Circle

Before screens and bedtime, sit in a circle (even on couches) and each share one thing you appreciated that day—encouraging positive focus and closing the day on a warm note.

Transition Rituals for Stressful Periods

Homework Huddle

At a set time (e.g., 6 pm), gather at the kitchen table for a quick "HQ meeting": set timers, review assignments, and confirm snack plans. The ritual signals "work mode" in a supportive, collective context.

Screen-Time Shutdown

Ten minutes before agreed cutoff, announce "two-minute warning," play a consistent song or timer sound, and then do a physical reset (walk, stretch) together to transition to family time.

Weekly Connection Ceremonies

Sunday Planning & Reflection

Combine calendar review—sports, chores, outings—with a brief sharing circle: "One thing I hope for this week is…" and "One thing I want to let go of from last week is…"

Family Fun Night

Rotate who picks a low-pressure activity—board game, movie, simple cooking project. Maintaining unpredictability within the routine keeps engagement high.

Monthly "Growth Check" Ritual

Review Progress Journal

Gather journal entries or behavior logs and note three areas of improvement and one area to focus on next month.

Goal-Setting Ceremony

Each member writes a personal goal on a colored card and places it on a "Growth Tree" (a simple branch in a vase). Visualizing goals makes them tangible and shared.

Incorporating Celebrations into Rituals

Milestone Markers: When a family member achieves a significant goal—consistent regulation for two weeks or completing a big project—ring a small bell or light a candle to gather everyone for applause.

Ritual Reinforcement: Tie celebrations into established ceremonies: mention that milestone during the gratitude circle or growth check to integrate acknowledgment seamlessly.

Ritual Evolution and Teen Agency

Co-Creation Sessions

Quarterly, hold a "Ritual Review": what feels ritualistic, what feels stale, and what new practices would everyone like to try?

Teen-Led Ceremonies

Invite teens to design one ritual—perhaps bedtime yoga, a shared playlist for transitions, or a weekly digital detox hour—boosting ownership and relevance.

Flexible Fidelity

While consistency is key, allow for exceptions (vacations, celebrations) and then recommit to the structure upon return. Flexibility prevents rituals from feeling punitive.

Monitoring Ritual Health

Engagement Metrics: Note whether rituals happen on schedule and how participants respond—enthusiasm, groans, or indifference can signal needed tweaks.

Feedback Loops: Use a quick "thumbs up/down" vote at the end of each ceremony to gauge approval and gather suggestions.

When rituals and routines are woven seamlessly into daily life—anchoring mornings, evenings, weeks, and months—they create an enduring scaffold of safety and connection. In this structured yet adaptable framework, relapse into old patterns becomes less likely: habits of cooperation, reflection, and mutual support become the family's default, rather than the exception.

Chapter 12: Looking Ahead: Nurturing Independence

Adolescence is both a culmination and a beginning: the culmination of years of guided growth, and the beginning of full-fledged adult life. As your teen approaches the threshold of independence—driving, college applications, first jobs—your role naturally shifts from rule-setter to coach, ally, and sounding board. In this final chapter, we cast our gaze forward, exploring how to **gradually loosen boundaries responsibly**, **coach essential life skills**, and **foster a lifelong parent-child partnership** that endures beyond the teenage years.

We begin by examining the art of gradually loosening boundaries without leaving your teen unmoored. Effective boundary-loosening balances autonomy with safety, using data from behavior logs and regular check-ins to guide increments of freedom. You'll learn a staged approach—trial periods, clear criteria for success, natural consequences—and discover how to calibrate privileges to your teen's evolving maturity.

Next, we delve into coaching three core life skills—communication, problem-solving, and self-advocacy—that transform theoretical responsibility into practical competence. We'll outline hands-on exercises, from role-plays to real-world apprenticeships, that build confidence and independence. You'll see how to structure feedback, set real deadlines, and create safe "fail forward" moments where your teen can learn from mistakes under your supportive eye.

Finally, we consider how to sustain a parent-child partnership well into adulthood. As your teen grows up, the relationship ideally evolves from parent-driven guidance to mutual counsel between two independent adults. We'll map rituals and check-in rhythms for emerging adults—college students, apprentices, first-job holders—and highlight ways parents can respect privacy while remaining emotionally available.

Nurturing independence is not a one-time act but a continuous, adaptive process. Over the next three sections, you'll gain a concrete roadmap for releasing the reins with confidence, empowering your teen with essential life skills, and cementing a partnership that thrives long after childhood ends. Let's look ahead together, forging the bridge from adolescence into adulthood.

Gradually loosening boundaries responsibly

Transitioning from strict supervision to trusting autonomy demands a deliberate, phased approach. Abruptly removing all limits can overwhelm a teen still refining judgment; keeping rules too long can stifle growth. The key is to **loosen boundaries in calibrated steps**, using performance data and collaborative negotiation to ensure each expansion of freedom is matched by demonstrated responsibility.

Establishing a Baseline of Trust

Review Behavioral Data

Examine logs and check-in summaries for success streaks: punctual homework submission, respectful communication, safe driving habits.

Identify Core Non-Negotiables

Clarify which safety rules remain inviolable (seat-belt use, alcohol abstinence, emergency check-ins) and which can shift.

Designing a Phased Freedom Plan

Tiered Privileges

Create three levels of autonomy:

Level 1: Added small freedoms (e.g., extended weekend curfew by 15 minutes).

Level 2: Moderate autonomy (unsupervised outings within a defined radius).

Level 3: Advanced privileges (overnight trips, independent use of shared car).

Trial Periods

Assign each tier a 2–4-week pilot. During the trial, track adherence to agreements and revisit weekly.

Clear Success Criteria

Define what constitutes "passing" each trial: no curfew violations, honest reporting of whereabouts, responsible spending.

Built-In Checkpoints

End each phase with a formal check-in: review data, discuss challenges, and decide together whether to advance, repeat, or adjust the trial.

Negotiating Adjustments

Collaborative Discussions

Frame each expansion as a negotiation: "You've shown consistent responsibility; what additional freedom feels appropriate?"

Conditional Offers

Use "if-then" proposals: "If you maintain a 95% on-time record for two weeks, then you can drive to the concert with friends."

Natural and Logical Consequences

Tie misuse of privileges directly to consequences: missing curfew results in reverting to the prior tier, not outright punishment.

Supporting Responsibility

Skill Check-Ins

Confirm your teen knows essential procedures: reading a map, checking gas levels, texting arrival times.

Resource Provision

Ensure they have necessary tools: a reliable phone, emergency contacts saved, and road-safety knowledge.

Parent Oversight Mechanisms

Implement minimal monitoring—shared calendar entries, geolocation "check-in" apps, group chats—to maintain connection without micromanagement.

Iterating and Refining

Data-Driven Tweaks

Use weekly logs to spot emerging issues (e.g., late-night texting shows fatigue). Adjust boundaries responsively.

Regular Reflection

Encourage your teen to self-evaluate: "How did this extra freedom feel? What challenges did you face?"

Celebrate Milestones

Mark each successful transition with acknowledgment—a note, a small ritual—to reinforce growth.

By breaking freedom into measured stages, supported by clear criteria and collaborative refinement, you ensure that each new boundary shift is earned and sustainable. Responsible autonomy becomes not a gift handed down, but a joint achievement grounded in trust and capability.

Coaching Life Skills: Communication, Problem-Solving, Self-Advocacy

True independence depends not just on freedom from rules, but on mastery of essential life skills. **Communication**, **problem-solving**, and **self-advocacy** form the triad that empowers teens to navigate work, relationships, and higher-education challenges. Below is a structured program for embedding these skills into everyday teaching moments.

Communication Skills

Active Listening and Expression

Role-Play Drills: Simulate common adult scenarios—job interviews, roommate conflicts—where your teen practices listening, paraphrasing, and asking clarifying questions.

Feedback Loop: Offer immediate, specific feedback—"You used a neutral tone when disagreeing; that kept the conversation constructive."

Written Communication

Email Etiquette: Teach them to draft professional emails—clear subject lines, polite greetings, concise body, and proper sign-offs.

Text/Chat Boundaries: Discuss the difference between casual and formal tone, and the importance of response timeliness.

Problem-Solving Skills

Structured Problem-Solving Framework

Introduce the five-step model: Define the problem, brainstorm solutions, evaluate options, implement a plan, and review the outcome.

Use real issues—budgeting for college, planning group projects—as practice grounds.

Decision-Making Exercises

Pros-and-Cons Grids: For larger life choices (choosing courses, jobs), have the teen list benefits and drawbacks, then assess which factors matter most.

Worst-Case Scenario Planning: Discuss potential pitfalls of each option and contingency actions, reducing decision anxiety.

Self-Advocacy Skills

Identifying Needs and Rights

Teach teens to articulate what they need—academic accommodations, mental-health breaks, or accommodations in jobs.

Role-play conversations with teachers, employers, or landlords: making clear requests, framing them courteously, and negotiating mutually acceptable solutions.

Building Confidence

Small Wins Portfolio: Help your teen document successful advocacy moments—asking for extra clarification in class or negotiating a later shift at work—and review them to build self-efficacy.

Impromptu Challenge: Occasionally present a low-stakes advocacy scenario spontaneously—calling a store to correct an order—and debrief afterward.

Integrating Skills into Routine

Weekly Skill Focus

Dedicate each week to one skill area: Monday role-play, Wednesday real-world application, Friday reflection.

Cross-Skill Projects

Plan activities that require all three: organizing a small event (communication with vendors, problem-solving logistics, advocating for budget).

Mentorship and Modeling

Introduce your teen to trusted adults—family friends, coaches—who exemplify these skills and can offer additional perspectives.

Feedback and Reflection

Guided Journaling

Encourage teens to write brief entries after skill applications: what went well, what they'd change next time.

Parent Check-Ins

Use "sandwich feedback": start with praise, offer one area for improvement, end with encouragement.

Peer Review

If your teen is comfortable, have them request feedback from classmates or colleagues on communication clarity or problem-solving teamwork.

By systematically teaching and reinforcing communication, problem-solving, and self-advocacy, you equip your teen with a versatile toolkit for adult challenges. As these skills become second nature, independence transforms from hope into reality.

Fostering a Lifelong Parent-Child Partnership

The parent-child relationship does not end when teens grow up; it evolves into a partnership of equals—two adults who once navigated childhood together. Cultivating this enduring alliance requires ongoing attention to **mutual respect**, **shared rituals**, and **adaptable support**. Below are strategies to lay the groundwork for a lifelong, resilient partnership.

Redefining Roles and Expectations

From Authority to Advisor

Gradually shift from directive guidance ("You must...") to consultative dialogue ("What are your thoughts on...?").

Updating Communication Norms

Establish adult-to-adult check-in preferences: frequency (monthly video call?), content (career goals, personal well-being), and boundaries (privacy around dating life).

Mutual Calendar Sharing

Maintain a shared digital calendar for significant events—graduation dates, family gatherings—ensuring both parties stay informed without overstepping.

Sustaining Shared Rituals

Annual Traditions

Keep a yearly ritual—holiday bake-off, summer road trip, New Year's goal session—that both look forward to and plan together.

Monthly "State of the Union" Chats

Set aside a consistent time each month to discuss life updates, challenges, and plans. Rotate facilitation to keep both invested.

Interest-Based Connectors

Cultivate one shared hobby—cooking, hiking, book club—so regular collaboration continues beyond childhood.

Balancing Autonomy with Availability

Open-Door Invitation

Communicate explicit welcome: "I'm here if you ever want advice or just to talk."

Respecting Boundaries

Honor your adult child's privacy; avoid unsolicited advice unless asked. Use gentle inquiries—"Would you like my input?"—before diving in.

Crisis-Ready Support

Maintain clarity on your willingness to help during emergencies—financial, health, or emotional—while delineating agreed-upon protocols (loan terms, confidentiality).

Evolving Conflict Resolution

Adult Repair Talk

Continue using "I feel… when you… because…" in disagreements, modeling mature conflict-resolution.

Boundary Negotiation

Revisit any friction points—holiday schedules, living arrangements—with the collaborative problem-solving techniques your teen has already mastered.

Third-Party Mediation

When needed, engage a trusted family friend or counselor to facilitate sensitive discussions, just as a professional coach might for a workplace dispute.

Celebrating Milestones Together

Life Transitions

Honor achievements—graduation, new job, home purchase—with thoughtful celebrations that recognize both independence and family roots.

Shared Legacy Projects

Collaborate on a memory book, family recipe collection, or genealogy project that cements the bond across generations.

Charitable Endeavors

Partner on a community service initiative—volunteering, fundraising—to reinforce shared values and purpose.

Maintaining Growth Mindset in the Partnership

Joint Learning

Enroll together in workshops or classes—cooking, financial planning, or a foreign language—to keep the relationship vibrant and evolving.

Feedback Exchange

Invite your young adult to give you feedback on your parenting journey: what they valued, what they wish had been different, fostering mutual growth.

Future Visioning

Periodically discuss long-term hopes—retirement travel plans, family legacy goals—positioning you as co-architects of a shared future.

By embracing your child as a developing partner rather than a perpetual dependent, you unlock a new relational phase marked by respect, choice, and mutual support. The same empathic listening, problem-solving, and celebration practices you've honed now fuel a lifelong partnership—one that adapts, deepens, and flourishes as you navigate the many seasons of adult life together.

Epilogue

As you set aside this book, pause to acknowledge the extraordinary work you and your teen have undertaken. What began as a struggle for control has blossomed into a shared journey of understanding. You've learned to listen more deeply, to hold firm without holding grudges, and to celebrate every small step toward respect and self-regulation. Your adolescent, through trial and error, has begun to see themselves not as a perpetrator of conflict, but as a capable agent of change—armed with tools for managing emotions, repairing relationships, and making choices that honor both their own needs and those of your family.

Yet this milestone is not an ending, but a new beginning. The rhythms you've established—clear boundaries met with compassion, rituals of check-in and celebration, and collaborative problem-solving—will continue to evolve as your teen grows into adulthood. There will be fresh challenges: shifting social landscapes, academic pressures, and the wider responsibilities of independence. When old patterns threaten to resurface, return to the principles you've practiced: empathy paired with accountability, consistency paired with flexibility, and connection paired with autonomy. Each time you reaffirm these commitments, you fortify the bridge between you and your child.

Above all, carry forward a sense of optimism and shared purpose. Parenting an adolescent who has veered into abusive behavior requires courage, patience, and humility—but it also offers the profound gift of transformation. The trust you rebuild today lays the foundation for a lifelong partnership built on mutual respect. Trust that, armed with the strategies and insights you've gained, both you and your teen possess the resilience to navigate future storms. Together, you'll continue to learn, adapt, and grow—one boundary, one bridge, and one moment of understanding at a time.

Appendices

Sample Boundary Contract

Boundary Contract		
Family Member(s): *Parent(s):* _____ *Teen:* _____		
Effective Date: _[Date] *Review Date:* [Date]		

Behavior (What)	Expectation (How)	Consequence if Violated
1. No physical aggression (hitting, pushing)	Keep hands and feet to yourself at all times—even during arguments	Natural: Repair any damage; Imposed: 24-hour loss of screen privileges
2. No name-calling or threats	Speak without insults or intimidation	Natural: Write a sincere apology letter; Imposed: Extra chores (1 hour per insult)
3. Curfew adherence	Be home by [time]; text if running late more than 10 minutes	Lost privileges: each unexcused late arrival = one evening grounded
4. Responsible digital use	No harassing texts, social-media tagging, or sharing private content without consent	Imposed: Social-media blackout for 48 hours; Natural: Apologize publicly if harm caused
5. Respectful communication	Use "I feel… when you… because…" before discussing disagreements	Imposed: Family meeting to practice communication scripts; Natural: Role-play apology

Signatures

Parent(s): _____ Date: _____

Teen: _____ Date: _____

Sample Behavior Chart

Use this chart daily (or weekly) to log incidents, note triggers, track consequences, and reflect on progress.

Date	Behavior Observed	Trigger / Context	Consequence Applied	Teen's Reflection (1–2 sentences)	Parent's Note (Progress or Concern)
2025 05 01	Yelled, "You're always against me"	Argument over chores after school	1 hour extra chores	"I felt attacked when asked to do dishes"	Took accountability; used breathing before next conflict
2025 05 02	Threw phone in anger	Denied extra screen time	Phone repair delay; apology note	"I overreacted; need to ask instead of smashing"	Phone intact; teen apologized without prompt
2025 05 03	Text-harassment of sibling	Jealous of sibling's success	48-hour social-media blackout	"I hurt my sister's feelings; sorry"	Sibling accepted apology; no repeat incident
2025 05 04	Stayed calm, used "I feel" script	Discussion about weekend plans	None	"I felt heard when we talked calmly"	Noted as a win —parent praise given

How to Use These Templates

Customize

Adjust behaviors, expectations, and consequences to fit your family's needs and your teen's age.

Collaborate

161

Fill out the contract and chart together so your teen has ownership.

Review Regularly

Post the contract in a common area; update the behavior chart daily or weekly and discuss patterns during your family check-ins.

These tools will help turn abstract goals into concrete agreements and actionable data—making it easier to maintain momentum, celebrate growth, and course-correct quickly when needed.

De-escalation Scripts

The Pause Signal

Parent: (Calmly holds up open hand) "I see things are heating up. Let's both take three deep breaths before we continue."

Teen: (Pauses, breathes) "Okay… I'm still upset, but I can talk."

Reflect-and-Redirect

Parent: "You sound really frustrated right now. Help me understand what's bugging you most."

Teen: "I just feel like you never listen!"

Parent: "I'm sorry you feel unheard. Let's slow down so I can listen better—what's one thing I might have missed?"

Choice Within Limits

Parent: "I can see we're both upset. Would you prefer to talk in the living room now, or take ten minutes in your room and reconvene here?"

Teen: "I'd like to cool off first."

Parent: "Great. Let's agree to come back in ten minutes and try again."

Calm Assurance

Parent: (Neutral tone) "I care about you and want to help. Let's lower our voices so we don't hurt each other—and figure this out together."

"Repair Talk" Templates

Use these sentence frames to name the rupture, own your feelings, and invite collaboration on next steps. Fill in the blanks together or model one for your teen.

Basic Repair

"I feel **[emotion]** when you **[action]** because **[impact]**, and I'd like us to **[desired change]**."

Example: "I feel worried when you slam the door because it makes me think you're more upset than you let on, and I'd like us to use words instead of slamming so we both feel heard."

Two-Step Repair

Acknowledge: "I realize I **[your behavior]**, and I'm sorry."

Request: "Next time, could you **[teen behavior request]** so we can avoid this?"

Example: "I realize I was late picking you up and didn't call—sorry about that. Next time, could you text me once you're done so you're not left waiting?"

Mutual Repair

Parent: "I feel **[emotion]** when I **[parent action]**, and you feel **[teen emotion]** when you **[teen action]**. Let's agree that next time we'll **[joint solution]**."

Example: "I feel rushed when I ask you to get ready right before we leave, and you feel cornered when I hurry you. Let's agree to start getting ready ten minutes earlier so neither of us feels stressed."

Future-Focused Repair

"Last time, when **[past incident]**, we both got upset. How about next time we try **[new strategy]**?"

Example: "Last time, when you yelled at me about chores, we both ended up angry. How about next time we use our 'pause and breathe' signal before talking about it?"

Tips for Both Scripts & Templates

• Practice these together during calm moments so they become second nature.

• Keep your tone gentle and body language open—repair is about reconnection, not blame.

• Write your chosen templates on a card or poster where you can both see them as reminders.

165

Resource list: books, websites, hotlines

Books

The Whole-Brain Child by Daniel J. Siegel & Tina Payne Bryson

Practical strategies for understanding and guiding developing brains.

Parenting from the Inside Out by Daniel J. Siegel & Mary Hartzell

Explores how parents' own experiences shape their parenting and offers tools for mindful connection.

No-Drama Discipline by Daniel J. Siegel & Tina Payne Bryson

A compassionate approach to setting limits and resolving conflicts without escalation.

The Explosive Child by Ross W. Greene

Introduces Collaborative & Proactive Solutions for challenging behaviour.

Trauma Through a Child's Eyes by Peter A. Levine & Maggie Kline

Insight into how trauma affects children and teens, with healing-focused exercises.

Websites

Child Mind Institute

childmind.org
Evidence-based guides on teen behavior, mental health, and parenting strategies.

The National Child Traumatic Stress Network

nctsn.org

Resources on trauma, self-help worksheets, and directories for local treatment centers.

Positive Parenting Solutions

positiveparentingsolutions.com

Online courses and free webinars on boundary setting, communication, and behavior management.

Aha! Parenting

ahaparenting.com

Dr. Laura Markham's blog offers empathetic parenting tips and downloadable guides.

How to Talk So Kids Will Listen & Listen So Kids Will Talk

howtotalk2kids.com

Companion site with exercises from the classic communication book by Faber & Mazlish.

Hotlines

Samaritans (UK & Ireland)

24/7 emotional support: 116 123

https://www.samaritans.org

Childline (UK)

Free, confidential support for young people under 19: 0800 1111

https://www.childline.org.uk

National Domestic Violence Hotline (US)

24/7 confidential support: 1-800-799-SAFE (7233)

https://www.thehotline.org

Crisis Text Line (US & Canada)

Text HOME to 741741 for free 24/7 support

https://www.crisistextline.org

Lifeline (Australia)

24/7 crisis support: 13 11 14

https://www.lifeline.org.au

Feel free to explore these resources for additional strategies, support networks, and professional referrals as you and your family continue on the path toward safety, healing, and reconnection.

Letter to My Readers

Dear Reader,

Thank you for joining me on this journey through ***Boundaries & Bridges: Parenting Strategies for Abusive Adolescents***. Writing this book has been both a professional endeavor and a deeply personal commitment—one born out of my experiences as a clinician, a mother, and an advocate for families in crisis. My hope is that these pages have offered you practical tools, compassionate insights, and renewed confidence as you navigate the challenges of parenting a teen whose behavior has crossed into harm.

Parenting an abusive adolescent can feel isolating, but you are not alone. Whether you're just beginning to set boundaries or you've been working toward healing for some time, remember that progress often comes in small, sometimes imperceptible steps. Celebrate the moments when your teen pauses to listen, when a tense conversation ends in apology rather than escalation, and when your home feels a little more peaceful. These are the milestones that mark real change.

I encourage you to stay in touch—your feedback, questions, and stories of transformation inspire me and help shape future resources. You can reach me via:

E-mail: AnissaBrodon@gmail.com
Amazon Author Page: https://shorturl.at/xwd82
Facebook: https://shorturl.at/O2gAn
Instagram: @AnissaBrodon
TikTok: @anissabrodon

Thank you for trusting me to walk alongside you. Together, we're building homes where safety and respect pave the way to healing and deeper connection. I look forward to hearing about your successes, learning from your challenges, and continuing this vital work—one boundary and one bridge at a time.

   With gratitude and hope,
Anissa Brodon

Index